THE CIRCLE OF LIFE

THE
CIRCLE OF LIFE

*A Search for an Attitude to Pain,
Disease, Old Age and Death*

by

KENNETH WALKER

'But he that is wisest amongst you is but a
discord, a hybrid of plant and ghost.'
Thus Spake Zarathustra
— NIETZSCHE

McGrath Publishing Company
College Park, Maryland

1970

Reprinted by
McGrath Publishing Co., 1970

ISBN: 0-8434-0072-2
LC # 76-119250

Reproduced from an original copy lent by
The University of North Carolina Library
at Chapel Hill

Manufactured in the United States of America
by Arno Press Inc., New York

CONTENTS

PREFACE

THE fact that many problems are insoluble does not prevent us from attempting to solve them. During many years of practice as a surgeon I have been collecting material out of which some sort of medical philosophy could be made. Not that I have given that title to the book which has eventually resulted. The word philosophy is liable to frighten the ordinary reader. It brings to his mind the disputations of the professional philosophers, the wordy warfare of dialecticians, the appeal of the learned to classical schools of thought and the nimble acrobatics of logic. But it is not in this sense that I would have used the word philosophy had I dared to place it on my title-page, but more in the sense in which it was used by Corin in *As You Like It* when he asked, 'Hast any philosophy in thee, shepherd?' or by Hamlet in speaking to Horatio. Aristotle came nearer to this when he wrote that philosophy is the product of wonder. As children we are all philosophers seeking from our elders explanations of the mysteries which surround us, wide-eyed with wonder and avid for knowledge. But the novelty of existence soon fades and by the time we have become adults most of us have lost all sense of wonder. Life has become for us a habit and, hypnotized by the preoccupations of wage-earning, sport and the routine of living, we cease to ask questions. Philosophy has become for us a study for a few leisured students who are freed from the necessity of earning a living. It is a matter for experts.

In a former work I attempted the difficult task of investigating the complex nature of man. In this book I have submitted to examination the ills to which man is subject. What is the meaning of the phenomena with which, as a doctor, I have become so familiar, illness and pain, fear, old age and death? Although no complete answer can be found for any of these questions, they are so closely woven into the fabric of our existence that they demand some explanation. This I have attempted to give. And because man is more than a biological unit, a mind and spirit as well as a body, the search for the meaning of man's sufferings has led me to deal with subjects which lie outside the realm of medicine. By doing so I have rendered myself vulnerable to the criticisms of the professional philosophers and expert metaphysicians. But I am not writing for the expert, but for the ordinary man and woman who still retain the capacity to wonder and to speculate about the mystery of existence.

Harley Street, W.1
1942

PART ONE

CHAPTER I

THE NEED FOR A PHILOSOPHY OF PAIN AND SUFFERING

THE existence of suffering in the world has long puzzled those who look to religious teachings for guidance. How can man's inheritance of pain and disease be reconciled with the rule of an Omnipotent, Omniscient and Compassionate Deity? To this question all the great leaders of world religions have given some answer which their followers have accepted with varying degrees of conviction. But there are many who, because they are unable to accept the authority of religion, have turned to science for an explanation. And no explanation has been given to them, for science is concerned only with the relationship existing between phenomena, and not 'with values and meaning. If a scientist does return an answer to the question: 'What is the meaning of illness and pain?' he speaks not as a scientist, but as a philosopher. Usually he prefers to remain silent, for scientists, as a class, are averse to philosophical speculation. If philosophy be 'the soul's adventure in the universe', then it must be confessed that neither scientists nor doctors show any liking for such adventure. They prefer to confine their attention to what they consider to be the more practical problems of their profession, and to leave to others the activity known to the Chinese as 'the thinking of thoughts afar off'. The disinclination of the doctor to speak of what does not appear to have any direct bearing on his work is easily understood. Doctors are so engrossed with the struggle against disease and suffering that they have no time to wonder how these phenomena fit into some larger whole. They are too near to their subjects to be able to see them in perspective, too preoccupied with urgent problems to deal with wider issues. In short, doctors are not called upon to develop a philosophy of disease, but to cure it.

Yet there is need of such a philosophy, and if it were available it would be of more than academic interest. We can accept better what we understand, and it is the meaninglessness of illness and pain which arouses our resentment. They appear to us to have erupted into a world which, though by no means ideal, would have been passable had it not been for their intrusion. Having no right to be there, we refuse to come to terms with them, or if, as sooner or later happens, we are forced to accept their presence, we do so grudgingly, feeling that we have been imposed upon, humiliated and insulted. But we are wrong in our original assumption that illness and pain are intruders in the circle of existence in which we move. They are the inevitable result of the conditions under which we live, and must be accepted as unreservedly as we accept the fundamental realities of birth and death. In order that we may attain this acceptance it is necessary to reach a better understanding of the nature of illness, pain and suffering, and, if such be attainable, of the still greater enigma of death.

And if a philosophy of illness, pain and suffering be necessary, who is in a better position to gather together the material out of which it can be made than the man who spends his life dealing with these things? Painters have glimpsed truth through their art and musicians through their music. May not a medical man through the experiences of the consulting-room reach some wider understanding of disease and pain? If illness is what a doctor understands best, then this should be the point from which he sets out in his search for deeper knowledge. He may be unversed in dialectics and have made no study of logic, but he starts with the initial advantage that he is acquainted with the instruments by which knowledge is gained, the intellect, the emotions and the special senses. To discover the unknown one must start from what one knows best, and by training and experience the medical man has become an expert in disease. This then should be his point of departure in his search for greater truths.

Before we can hope to discover the meaning of disease, we must first arrive at some understanding of its nature. Complaint has frequently been made that doctors cannot define what they spend their lives treating. This is not strictly true, for many definitions of disease have been provided, each one embodying the medical ideas of the age in which it was formulated. Because medicine is an art resting on a scientific basis, these different definitions of disease reflect the changing views of science. Thus in Judea at the time of Christ, disease was defined in terms of possession by an evil spirit, in Europe in the time of Galen, it was held to be a disturbance of the four cardinal humours of the body, and subsequent to Pasteur's epoch-making discoveries, illness was attributed to the invasion of the body by hostile micro-organisms. Because science never reaches finality the basis of medicine is continually shifting and medical definitions have to be periodically amended. This adjustment of medical definitions to changes of scientific theory has had to be made during the course of the last fifty years and it will be necessary to describe briefly the repercussion of science on contemporary medicine.

The Victorian scientists interpreted everything in the universe in terms of mechanism, and as a direct result of this, the doctors of that age looked upon a sick man as a machine which had suffered some breakage; something had gone wrong with the patient's structure, and the wheels of his being no longer ran smoothly. With the growth of pathology a more exact account of the breakage in mechanism could be given; a man was ill because the working of the liver was faulty, because the bowel was obstructed, or because the valves of the heart had been damaged. This greater precision in diagnosis brought with it many advantages, but it was also fraught with a new danger. The identification of illness with a badly working organ inevitably led to a shifting of the physician's attention from the patient as a whole to that part of him which seemed to be most affected. Doctors became so engrossed in the treatment of an enlarged liver, an obstructed bowel or defective heart valve that they were in grave danger of forgetting the existence of a sentient and suffering patient. This limited conception of illness was unfortunate, for a man is something more than a number of organs cleverly packed together and surrounded by a waterproof wrapping. He is a living being possessed of a mind as well as of a body, a complex organism no part of which can be disturbed without the whole being affected. Growing specialization in medical practice increased the dangers resulting from this organ-conception of disease. Each organ of the body became an isolated field of study for a separate group of experts, who, not unnaturally, showed a tendency to view ill health in terms of their own particular speciality. Now whilst specialization was essential for the progress of medicine, it undoubtedly accentuated the errors resulting from the 'damaged organ' view of disease. All specialists are in a manner prejudiced, and look at patients through their own tinted glasses. Even when they work as a team, under the same roof, they cannot escape from their predilections. Team work has been brought to the highest level of efficiency in that world-famous centre of medicine, the Mayo Clinic of Rochester, U.S.A. Into this gigantic and superbly equipped health factory for many years has poured an unending stream of raw material, the halt, the sick and the maimed. Once within its portals they are (figuratively) caught up on a belt running on well-oiled machinery; they are weighed, measured, analysed, photographed, X-rayed, trans-illuminated, inspected, electro-cardiogrammed and meticulously tested. The Mayo Clinic is a true child of the United States of America, the home of mechanized, departmentalized, industrialized medicine raised to the highest degree of efficiency, and is worthy of the great home of mass-production and mechanized industry, of statistical surveys and Gallup polls. The results obtained by this famous Rochester institution have been magnificent, but sometimes underlying disadvantages are seen through the surface of efficiency. A patient, during his passage through the various departments of the Mayo Clinic, undoubtedly accumulates a vast amount of information concerning the working of his various organs, but when the examinations have been completed and the final notes added to his impressive 'dossier', little more may be known about the real nature of his illness than when he entered the Clinic's doors. In such cases, the synthesis of the various observations, measurements, indices and analytical records have proved too difficult even for the extremely efficient directors of the Clinic. The patient has been so completely taken to pieces that nobody is able to look upon him again as a whole being. He is no longer an individual man but a jumble of scientific data.

Fortunately we are now witnessing a reaction from this departmentalized and 'broken-machine' view of illness, just as we are witnessing a reaction from a mechanistic explanation of the universe. The change in the doctor's attitude to disease is partly the result of the scientists' new discoveries in the realm of physics. Matter has now been identified with energy and the scientist has repainted the picture by which he represents the universe. For space occupied by myriads of solid atoms he has substituted a space-time continuum disturbed by vibratory differentiations. Medicine obediently follows the lead given by the scientist, and since the scientist has substituted a dynamic for a static picture of the universe, so must the doctor now substitute a dynamic for a static view of life. He can no longer regard a sick man as a broken machine, but must look upon him as being an energy-system in which the balance of forces has been disturbed. An up-to-date definition of illness would, therefore, be to the effect that it is an upsetting of the equilibrium of an energy-system, by the impact of some hostile force. Disease is a state of disequilibrium.

But little satisfaction will be found in this, or, for that matter, in any other definition of illness. A search for definitions of fundamental concepts generally yields only meagre results. Can the lawyer define justice, or the theologians formulate in a few words what they mean by God? It is not only the doctor who finds difficulties in defining the concepts of his calling, and more will be gained from studying the nature of disease than from any further attempt to confine it within the boundaries of a definition. 'Definitions', declared the petulant Samuel Butler, 'are a kind of scratching and generally leave a sore place more sore than it was before.'

It is important to realize that the word 'disease' is used loosely by laymen, and often by doctors. At one time it is applied to the hostile agent, and at another to the disturbance which this provokes. When a man states that he has just recovered from an attack of scarlet fever, he generally has in mind the sore throat, the headache, the aches and pains, the rash and the high temperature from which he has recently suffered. But all these discomforts were but the outward signs of the resistance which his body was offering to the streptococci which had invaded it, and without these disturbances he would undoubtedly have succumbed to his infection. In that particular case a clear distinction can be drawn between the hostile agent and the body's reaction to it, but in the case of diabetes, where the cause is unknown, we are compelled to think of the illness in terms of the disturbances which it occasions. Consequently by diabetes we mean a combination of signs and symptoms — thirst, wasting, changes in the pancreas, and sugar in the urine. As we are generally more familiar with the reactions of the body during illness than with the actual cause of them, it is natural that we should identify most diseases with their symptoms rather than with their causes. This is particularly likely to be the case when the symptoms happen to be particularly violent, and the exciting cause comparatively insignificant. Asthma is a good example of a disease in which the symptoms are out of proportion to their cause. This complaint is characterized by a violent spasmodic contraction of the muscle fibres surrounding the bronchial tubes, a contraction which may be provoked in susceptible subjects by such trifling causes as pollen in the air, exertion, a mild attack of indigestion, or an emotional disturbance. It should be noted that what must be regarded as pathological in asthma is not the reaction of the bronchial muscles — this is a normal response — but its violence.

Asthma is only one example of a whole class of diseases characterized by an exaggerated response on the part of the organism to a comparatively insignificant stimulus. These illnesses are now grouped under the heading 'allergy', a condition of hypersensitiveness. For example, some individuals are born with an abnormal sensitiveness to a stimulus which has but little effect on their fellows; the application of turpentine to one person's skin will produce an acute dermatitis, whilst in others it only causes a slight reddening. Again, one person will suffer no ill effects from taking quinine, but another will react violently, developing headache, dizziness, ringing in the ears, and even a skin eruption. All these are examples of what is known as idiosyncrasy, that is to say, of an individual hypersensitiveness to a particular form of stimulus, and idiosyncrasy is the explanation of a certain type of illness. What is of particular interest from the point of view of the relationship between body and mind is that there exists a condition of hypersensitiveness of the mind as well as of hypersensitiveness of the body. As some people react excessively to a mild irritant, such as turpentine, so do some minds respond violently to a mild psychic disturbance. They live in a state of unstable equilibrium, their minds being 'allergic' to the mildest emotional disturbances. In both instances the nature of the trouble is the same, namely, an excessive response of the body or of the mind to a comparatively weak stimulus. Frequently a patient who exhibits a hypersensitiveness to physical stimuli shows an excessive emotional response to a trifling psychic irritant, thus lending support to the view that mind and body are but different aspects of a single entity.

The nature of illness, whether it be psychic or somatic, is therefore

14

essentially the same; it is a disturbance in the balance of the complicated energy-system which we call life. In many cases the disturbance starts as a conflict between the forces within the organism and those which surround it, and ends with an upset in the balance maintained between the various parts of the organism. The great differentiation of structure which has taken place in the higher forms of life carries with it certain grave disadvantages. It demands the maintenance of a nice balance between the different parts, and thus becomes a potential source of weakness. Should the inner harmony be disturbed by any of the accidents to which all individual organisms are subjected, one set of organs is weakened in relation to the others, and thus produces illness. Just as complicated instruments are more often in need of repair than are simple instruments, so are highly differentiated organisms more liable to become ill than are simpler organisms. Looked at from this angle illness is an accident to which all energy-systems are subject, and more particularly the highly unstable energy-systems of the higher organisms.

A human being is the most complicated of all living things and the most susceptible to disturbances of that inner harmony which we call health. Man is subject to discords of which the animal knows nothing, to the strife of the spirit as well as to the turmoil of the body. And since mind and body are so interdependent as to be inseparable, disturbances on one plane of man's existence are quickly communicated to the other. An illness which starts with an emotional conflict ends with physical disharmony, a faulty adjustment of the body leads to psychic distress. It is not man's body or his mind but the whole of his being which reacts to the disturbances to which he is subject.

In a recent book Guirdham has called attention to the important part played by strain in the genesis of illness. He states that we can trace five stages in the development of many diseases: strain, anxiety, postural defect, functional disturbance, and finally structural changes. He then somewhat pessimistically remarks: 'The function of present day medicine is largely to patch up patients for a speedy return to an illogical civilization, which will continue to break them down.' The author of *Disease and the Social System* may have attributed too much blame to our civilization in the production of disease, but it is impossible to exaggerate the importance of the factor of strain. It has long been known that certain lesions, such as writer's cramp, housemaid's knee, tennis elbow and miner's nystagmus are the direct result of the excessive strain imposed on certain structures by certain occupations, but it has only comparatively recently been realized that the increase during the last fifty years of diseases of the central nervous system is attributable to the stresses of modern civilized life. There has been a rise in the incidence not only of such functional disorders as neurasthenia and various forms of neuroses, but also of organic diseases affecting the central nervous system, disseminated sclerosis, infantile paralysis, encephalitis, cerebral spinal fever, and even cerebral tumour. It is the central nervous system which receives the first impact of the weight of modern life, and it is in this structure that doctors frequently find the earlier signs of many illnesses.

Disease has been described as a disharmony of the whole inner organism which has been brought about by its failure to adjust to an external strain. One point is in need of clarification before proceeding further. It should be noted that when health is stated to be a condition of equilibrium in a complex system of forces, the word equilibrium is not used in the same sense as it is in physics and chemistry. Life was once defined by Lapicque as a struggle against physical laws, and by Claude Bernard as 'a combination of functions which resist death'. It entails endless adjustment and struggle, and never for one moment can the forces within a living creature remain in a state of quiet. Change is the very essence of living and only with death does the body attain the degree of immobility possessed by inert matter. The equilibrium of life is an equilibrium which is continually in need of readjustment.

Man seeks to find some significance in the disturbances to which his person is subjected. It is not sufficient for him to know that he shares with all around him a precarious and insecure existence, but he seeks to discover some advantage hidden under the apparent evil of disease. He is wishful in his thinking and many attempts have been made by scientists, by artists, and by leaders of religion to find a purpose which is useful to man in the existence of human illness. Biologists have, for example, suggested that it may be a means of weeding out physical weakness and of thus improving the stock. But even if we accept Darwin's theory of Natural Selection — and there is much to be said against it — it is extremely doubtful whether disease can be looked upon as being a means of eliminating the unfit. In Sir Humphrey Rolleston's words:

> Many besides the degenerate fall victims, and disease which has been at work and on its trial in this respect from, or before, the dawn of history is too rough and unorganized a method to bring about the survival of the fittest.

With this I am in full agreement, for whilst it is true that an epidemic of influenza sweeps away many idiots and weaklings, it takes at the same time a large toll of the intelligent and fit. Disease is too lacking in discrimination to be regarded as a satisfactory collaborator of the eugenist. It is impossible to look upon it as Nature's method of improving the quality of the stock. That sadly overworked slogan, 'the survival of the fittest', cannot be used in this connection; and since this is the answer which the biologist usually offers when confronted with a difficult question, we can assume that the biologist is unable to enlighten us as to the function of disease.

The effort of artists and writers to find some meaning in disease is equally unsatisfactory. It has often been said and written that many of the greatest achievements in literature and art must be credited to men of indifferent health, who, because they have been denied physical well-being, have devoted all their energies to the cultivation of the mind, and by their work have conferred lasting benefits on humanity. This is undoubtedly true. So also are Goethe's words to Eckermann true. In speaking of the ill health of men of creative achievement ability he remarked:

> Their extraordinary achievement presupposes a very delicate organization which makes them susceptible to unusual emotions and capable of hearing celestial voices. Such an organization, in conflict with the world and the elements, is easily disturbed and injured; he who does not, like Voltaire, combine with great sensibility an equally uncommon toughness, is liable to constant illness. Schiller was always ill. When I first knew him, I thought he could never live a month; but he too had a certain toughness; he kept going for many years, and would have done so longer if he had lived in a healthier way.

But some have gone even further than Goethe and have asserted that the work done by an ailing artist gains some new quality from its

creator's ill health. For example, it is often stated that much of
R. L. Stevenson's best writing was done during bouts of fever, and
that Nietzsche and Maupassant produced masterpieces while in the
early stages of the disease from which they eventually died. But an
argument based on a few selected and exceptional cases is wholly un-
scientific, for it is quite impossible to judge what such men might have
achieved if they had remained healthy. In all probability literature and
art have lost more than they have gained through the illness of their
creators. Keats has left us some of the loveliest poetry in the English
language, but his early death from phthisis deprived us of the work
of the maturer man. Carlyle's poor digestion may have introduced an
irascible note into his writing, but it was in no way responsible for his
genius. Byron's club-foot rendered him over-sensitive, with all that
this implies, and at the same time it may have been responsible for the
uneven quality of his verse. Whilst physical handicaps have undoubtedly induced certain individuals to find compensation in the
sphere of the mind, they have never converted an indifferent into a
brilliant writer, or an incompetent into a competent artist. We have it
from Nietzsche himself that ill health made him into a philosopher,
but it is not to ill health but to his genius that must be accorded the
brilliance of *Thus Spake Zarathustra*.

All these attempts to find a meaning and purpose in illness suffer
from the defect that they view it only from the standpoint of the
individual man. If we are to find an answer to the question: 'What is
the function and the meaning of disease?' we must widen the scope of
our inquiry, and consider disease not only from the standpoint of
man but from the ampler viewpoint of life on the earth. Man is not
the only inhabitant of this planet. He is one of many living creatures,
a single constituent of the complex circle of life which encompasses
the earth, and penetrates into its outermost layers. Only after we have
examined the large-scale phenomena of the total aggregate of life
in which man has his being will it be possible to obtain more understanding of the meaning of disease.

CHAPTER II

THE CIRCLE OF LIFE ON THE EARTH

ALTHOUGH inconsistency is anathema to the scientist, the scientific account of the appearance of life on this planet contains strange inconsistencies. When an astronomer describes the earth, he refers slightingly to it as one of the minor planets revolving round a star of the second magnitude. If pressed to account for the appearance of life upon it, he tells us that owing to a unique concatenation of circumstances, and at a certain stage of the earth's cooling, certain large molecules came together, became organized and developed the properties of life. And then after the course of millions of years another astounding accident happened: part of this mildew covering the earth became conscious. Man, sentient and restless, appeared, man the seeker after truth, man, creation's brilliant afterthought, man who demanded some explanation of his presence in this remote corner of a vast empty universe. And he has good reason to be puzzled by the astronomer's story of his birth. If, as they tell him, here only in the whole of creation dwell living and conscious beings, then a splendid miracle has happened, a miracle which has raised an insignificant planet high above the empty splendour of the stars. If only here exist consciousness and life, then this poor earth has become pre-eminent in the universe. No longer can it be regarded as an insignificant planet but rather as a single oasis of conscious life in a dead, uninhabited desert of stars.

Fortunately it is not necessary for our present purposes either to accept or to reject this unconvincing story told by the scientists. Whether only on this earth have appeared intelligent beings, or whether they exist elsewhere, is at the moment immaterial to us. We need only start with the fact that life exists on this planet, and that it is so ubiquitous as to cover its surface with a film which, for all practical purposes, may be regarded as being continuous. This continuity is not apparent to us, for we see only those forms of life which have attained certain dimensions and are visible to the naked eye. We are conscious of the existence of our fellow-men, of animals, of insects, of trees and grass, but not of the tiny creatures, the minute unicellular organisms, and the various forms of bacteria which form the bulk of the earth's inhabitants. And by continuity is meant not merely a space relationship but an uninterrupted sequence of life processes. As the notion of isolated particles of matter has proved untenable in physics, so also will the idea of self-contained organisms, living as self-sufficient beings within their local habitations, prove unsatisfactory in biology. Life on this earth is continuous in more senses than that it is so prolific as to be almost in contact; it is continuous also in the sense that the life processes of different organisms are complementary and interdependent.

When as a child I escaped from some petty domestic difficulty, on to the hillside, or into a wood, I always had the feeling that I was not alone. Human beings had been left behind in the house, but here on the hill, or in the wood, there was a mighty presence, serene, understanding and all-powerful. In some way I was part of this great being to which I had fled, and it accepted my presence as natural. I felt comforted, and, at the same time, a little awed. The presence was not the all-powerful, all-seeing God which the Sunday school spoke about, but something which was much closer, more intimate and more akin to myself. An air of expectation hung over the wood, and I felt that if I were to lie quiet and listen, perhaps some sign would be given to me, and I would discover the great mystery of life. This feeling of being part of a great life, this sense of kinship with all that moves and breathes and grows upon the earth, has been described by many of our great writers, and notably by W. H. Hudson. Hudson writes of those vivid moments in which he felt the nearness of some great presence which he calls Nature. But this word does not satisfy me. Nature is too big and would have included everything in those childish experiences on the hillside or in the wood, from the stones at my feet to the blue line of hills in the distance. The presence which I sensed as a boy was more nearly related to me, and closer. It was life, not individualized living, but life as a whole, life in the trees, in the undergrowth, in the grass on which I sat, in the rich earth into which I dug my fingers. I was part of the great life which breathed and throbbed and lay around me.

Lotze, the philosopher, has said of any philosophical system that it is 'an attempt to justify a fundamental view of things which has been adopted early in life'. I believe this to be true, and that the nature of the philosophy which a mature man reaches is to a great extent predetermined by the quality of his emotions in childhood and in youth. And philosophy is as much a product of the emotions as of the intellect. Truth is not reached through the throbbing of a few fibres in an elderly philosopher's brain, but by the whole of a man's faculties working to one end. The intellect confirms and gives an outline to what the emotions with their bigger sweep into the unknown have discovered; it formulates and renders communicable what previously was only felt. As a child I sensed the unity of all life; as a man I discovered intellectual arguments to support what before was only unformulated feeling. Slowly, as the mind works upon it, a new concept begins to take shape; connections are made with other concepts, and in time a new belief finds its place, not only in the heart, but also in the head. Then comes ratification from reading, and what had at one time seemed to be a personal discovery is found to be perhaps a widely accepted belief. Thus is evolved a philosophy, or as Lotze would say, the justification of 'a fundamental view of things which has been adopted early in life'.

Organic life on the earth forms an integrated whole, and it is only by relating the individual to the mighty organism in which he lives that such problems as birth, disease, old age and death can be understood. J. B. S. Haldane repeatedly lays stress on this relating of the part to the whole in his book, *Mechanism, Life and Personality*:

> In normal reproduction and death, and in all instinctive and social activity, the individual organism shows itself to be more than an individual; it belongs to a wider organic whole, apart from which most of its life is unintelligible.

Haldane compares the separate organisms existing in organic life to the cells out of which the body is built up, and the analogy is a close one. Just as a balance is maintained between the various kinds of cell in the body, so does there exist an equilibrium between the many types of separate organisms found in the sum total of organic life on the earth. Isolated from its neighbours and grown in a culture tube, a fragment of tissue will grow almost indefinitely, but situated in the body and hemmed in by other tissues, the growth of these cells is limited. Each variety of tissue in the body exerts an inhibitory action on the growth of its neighbour, the balance maintained by all conforming to the needs of the organism. The same is true of the sum total of organic life on the earth. Within this great aggregate there exists an infinite number of different organisms, some of them differing so profoundly in structure and in method of living as to have only one characteristic in common with their fellows, namely that they are alive and form part of organic life. Yet the relationship between these seemingly incongruous elements is so nicely adjusted that they not only contrive to live together, but even create the illusion of having an independent existence. That the independence is an illusion is certain, for each component of the Great Life lives only through and by means of the other. Were one of the three great sections of organic life — animals, vegetables and micro-organisms — to be eliminated, the whole finely balanced structure would fall in ruins, like a groined roof deprived of the support of its essential arches. It is, of course, obvious that if all vegetation were to disappear from the earth, the whole of the animal kingdom would die. But what would appear to be a much less important change than this would be equally disastrous. It can be shown that the elimination of micro-organisms, the unseen component of organic life, would be sufficient to cause the ruin of all. Since micro-organisms are responsible for the majority of diseases, and at the same time are essential to the well-being of organic life, they are of particular interest to us at the present moment. It will be necessary to consider them in greater detail.

Before discussing micro-organisms in general, it must be pointed out that those responsible for disease constitute only a small minority in the world of bacteria. The bad reputation of this comparatively unimportant group has given rise to the popular misconception that micro-organisms in general are the hereditary enemies of man. This is the exact reverse of the truth. Generally speaking, the activities of micro-organisms are in the highest degree beneficial to the human race. Indeed, a world devoid of bacteria would be a world in which man could not live. It would be almost as uninhabitable as would be a world without water, for micro-organisms occupy in the biological sphere a position which is as important as is that of water in the physical sphere. As water is found everywhere, so also are micro-organisms found in the earth beneath our feet, in the air that we breathe, in the food that we consume and in the tissues of which we are made. They and we are bound together in a lifelong partnership, a partnership which even survives death, for decomposition is carried out by means of the ceaseless activities of bacteria.

No better example could be given of the debt which we owe to the unseen organisms around us than that supplied by a study of the bio-chemistry of nitrogen. This will be summarized briefly and with the use of as few technical terms as possible. It must be realized that the protoplasm which enters largely into the structure of our bodies, and which has been looked upon as being the physical basis of life, is an exceedingly complex material. It is built up from the proteins which are a necessary ingredient of our food, and which are dis-tinguished from the two other essential foods, namely, carbohydrates and fats, by their containing nitrogen as well as carbon, hydrogen and oxygen. The proteins which we require in order to maintain the structure of our bodies can be obtained from both animal and vegetable food. But whether we be meat eaters or vegetarians is of little account, for in either case the proteins have in the first place been derived from the vegetable world. What is true of us is equally true of all animals. Sometimes the vegetable source of protein from which an animal re-plenishes his body is consumed directly, as in the case of a cow, and sometimes it is separated from the animal consumer by several stages, as in the somewhat complicated example furnished by F. M. Burnet in his book, *Biological Aspects of Infectious Diseases*:

> A shark feeds on large fish which in most cases capture smaller fish. These probably find their main food supply in small crus-taceans, which feed on the protozoa of the surface waters. The protozoa live on microscopic green algae, the unicellular plant organisms, which are the final source of food of most marine animals.

Vegetation is, therefore, the original source of all our nitrogenous foods, and but for the existence of plants on the earth, animal life would perish. Now, although a small proportion of our nitrogenous food is built up into our bodies to make good wear and tear, the greater part of it is used only as fuel. Fuel, whether it be that of the body, or of an engine, liberates energy in the course of being broken down into simpler compounds or waste products. In the case of the protein fuel under consideration the waste products to which it gives rise are urea and uric acids, which are excreted in the urine, and in this manner find their way back to the soil. The energy which is liberated in the breaking down of the proteins into urea and uric acid is manifested in the form of heat, muscular movements and in the numerous activities of the body.

It is important to realize that there is a fundamental difference in the life chemistry of animals and plants. Whereas animals resolve their food into simpler substances, plants work in the opposite direction, building up simple substances into more complex ones. Because their tastes are complementary, animals and plants, like Jack Spratt and his wife, live together in happy harmony. They are two well-balanced and mutually helpful components of organic life, living on each other and through each other. The difference in their chemistry renders them suitable partners and they may be looked upon as being symmetrical and complementary curves in the general pattern of life. A well-known instance of the plant's capacity to build up simple into complex molecules is its power to combine the carbon dioxide of the air with water, for the making of the starch, sugar and cellulose which enter so largely into their structure. This work of photo-synthesis is accomplished by the plant's green colouring matter, or chlorophyl, which utilizes the radiant energy of sunlight for building aldehyde out of carbon dioxide and water. The sun is therefore as essential to the life of the plant as is the earth on which it lives. Plants not only manufacture carbohydrates with the help of the sun's energy, but they also have the capacity to build up complex protein molecules out of the nitrates which they absorb from the soil. It is not benevolence, but necessity, which causes a plant to go to all this trouble of laboriously building up simple into complex substances. If some sentimental gardener were to supply a plant with the finished products instead of with the ingredients for making them, it would be unable to utilize them. Nature has ordained that a plant should start from the beginning with the simplest material and has forbidden to it all short cuts. Even the waste products returned by animals into the soil are too complex for its use. However rich the earth might be in urea and uric acid, vegetation would die unless it also contained the simpler substances which it needs, namely nitrates, and these can only be obtained by a further breaking down of animal waste products. Here, apparently, is a flaw in the partnership of animals and plants. Whilst animals can make full use of plants as food, plants cannot avail themselves of the nitrogenous waste products returned by animals into the soil. There exists, therefore, a gap between the form in which nitrogen is excreted by animals (urea and uric acid), and that in which it becomes serviceable to plants (nitrates), a gap which, unless it were bridged, would inevitably lead to a gradual impoverishment of the soil and an eventual disappearance of all vegetation. It is here that the third partner in the triangle of life, namely, bacteria, perform a service of vital importance to plants, and consequently, to all living creatures. The myriads of micro-organisms which live in the soil break down animal excreta into the simple substances required by vegetation; one class of bacteria reduces the urea to ammonia, another changes this into nitrites, and yet another finally converts the nitrites into nitrates. By this series of changes the nitrogenous waste products of the animals are metamorphosed into the nitrogenous food of plants. The vital gap in the nitrogen cycle has been bridged.

But chemists have shown us that this method of converting urea into nitrates is wasteful since in the process of change part of the nitrogen escapes into the air and is lost. Now life on the earth is run along strictly economical lines. If this wastage of nitrogen were not rectified, the soil in course of time would become impoverished. The remedy is again provided by micro-organisms, to be more precise by the nitrogen-fixing bacteria which live in the nodules found on the roots of certain leguminous plants. These organisms have the power of building up nitrates from free nitrogen. Because the so-called 'nitrogen-fixers' live in the roots of peas, clover, vetch and beans, farmers practise what is called the rotation of crops, sowing clover in a field after its soil has been impoverished by wheat. This has the same effect as covering the field with animal manure and is a cheaper method of replenishing the soil with nitrates.

It will be seen, therefore, that at two points in the nitrogen cycle, bacteria intervene in order to make life possible for both animals and vegetation; first, in converting animal excreta into food assimilable by plants, and second, in allowing them also to make use of free nitrogen in the air. Great though these services to life on the earth be they are not all that the bacteria perform. Sooner or later animals and plants die, and thus cease to be producers of nitrogenous excreta and builders up of proteins. But even though they be dead, their bodies contain a large amount of nitrogen which would be of great value to the soil if it could be liberated from the tissues. Again bacteria lend their services, and by bringing about putrefaction enrich the soil with the nitrates which it requires. Bacteria may therefore be said to be as essential to the life of the plant as the plant is to the life of the animal. Together these three components of organic life — animals, plants and bacteria — form a high arch on which rests the whole structure of life.

It would not be necessary for some criminal scientist, desirous of destroying humanity, to discover a means of exploding the atom. He could equally well achieve his purpose by devising a method of destroying bacteria. Bigger gives us a thumbnail sketch of what would happen should he succeed in doing this:

> Without bacteria, the nitrogen cycle would come to a full stop. The reserves of nitrates in the soil and in certain deposits, such as those of Chile, together with artificially produced nitrates, would permit of a sort of cultivation of crops for perhaps a couple of years, and then all growth of vegetation would cease. Next, the lower animals would die miserably of starvation, and then would come man's turn. A few might struggle on for a time on hoarded food, relic of the bacterial age, but starving millions would ferret out their supplies which, divided among many, would not last long. Very soon the last surviving man, emaciated, scurvy-ridden from the lack of fresh food, and no more fortunate because his body was free from all bacterial disease, would perish miserably, proving that the continued existence of all higher forms of life depends on the never-ceasing activities of the lowly bacteria.

Bacteria swarm in all dead organic material, and, as we have seen, are responsible for the processes of putrefaction and decay. Fortunately the micro-organisms which are responsible for these changes can only attack us after death. There are, however, bacteria living within us during life, bacteria which make use of the indigestible residues in our food as it passes along the lower bowel. So many different varieties of bacteria lodge within the large intestine that this part of our anatomy may be regarded as a battleground which reproduces in miniature the struggle for existence which we ourselves are waging on the surface of the earth. Similar bacterial conflicts are taking place on other surfaces of our bodies, in the mouth, throat and nose and in the outer layers of the skin. Not only do we suffer no inconvenience from the strife within us but our digestive processes even derive some benefit from it. A good example of a benefit conferred by bacteria living within an organism is provided by the termites. These creatures themselves are entirely unable to digest the wood and vegetable matter on which they live. This work is done for them by the cellulose-digesting bacteria living within them.

But we know to our cost that all bacteria are not equally well disposed towards us. As there are piratical and racketeering, as well as honest traders in a city, so may there be marauding, as well as benevolent bacteria in our bodies. When these gain the ascendancy we become ill; when the body has successfully mobilized its resistance and overcome them, we recover. It is generally supposed that the predatory or pathogenic (disease-carrying) bacteria have been evolved from harmless ancestors. According to this theory the struggle for existence among bacteria became so fierce that new subterfuges for survival had to be found. Instead of remaining satisfied with what sustenance the body provided for them in the way of indigestible residues of food and of cells cast off from mucous linings, certain organisms evolved a new method of livelihood by attacking the body's vast stores of living protoplasm. This predatory form of life was made possible by the organisms developing the power to form toxins, or poisons, which, by lowering the vitality of the host's body, prepared the way for invasion. The similarity that often exists between pathogenic organisms and the harmless bacteria which are normally found in the body supports the view that they are descended from the same ancestors. Thus the virulent bacilli of typhoid fever resemble so closely the coliform bacilli which normally inhabit the bowel, that the two can only be distinguished from each other by the use of special bacteriological tests. Similarly, the bacillus of diphtheria is almost identical with the harmless diphtheroids found in the healthy throat. This strongly suggests that typhoid and diphtheria bacilli are forms of coliform and diphtheroid bacteria which have evolved a new mode of life in order to survive. It must be admitted, however, that there are bacteriologists who do not accept this theory of the evolution of disease. They base their objection on the fact that the development of predatory habits does not always prove an advantage, and that sometimes it may defeat its own ends. For example, the vibrio of cholera is so virulent that it rapidly kills the host which sustains it and thus encompasses its own ruin. Only if the cholera vibrios can manage to establish a colony in a new host can the race survive the destruction of its whole world by the death of its host. The bacillus of tuberculosis would appear to be wiser in its behaviour, for by curbing its powers of destruction it contrives to live for many years in the same body, and, at the same time, provides itself with ample opportunities for establishing new colonies in other people. One man or animal therefore gives sustenance to tubercle bacilli for a period of many years, rather than, as is the case of the cholera vibrio, for only a few days. The disadvantages which result from bacteria being too virulent are so obvious that some bacteriologists regard the development of pathogenicity in micro-organisms as being an unfortunate accident, and not a method which has been evolved for the purpose of survival. In support of this view they cite the case of the bacillus of tetanus (lockjaw) which lives a happy and uneventful life in man's intestines without causing him any trouble. When, however, the tetanus bacillus forsakes its normal habitat and invades man's tissues, causing lockjaw, it signs its own, as well as its victim's, death warrant. The tetanus bacillus would obviously have been wiser to have remained sinless in the Eden in which Providence had placed it. By the eating of forbidden fruit it accomplishes its own ruin.

Although bacteria and viruses are not the sole agents of disease they are undoubtedly responsible for the majority of illnesses. No statistics can be given to indicate what percentage of illness is microbial in origin, if for no other reason than that the precise causes of many diseases still remain unknown to us. For example, we do not know the cause of cancer. Some experts believe that it is caused by an, as yet, undiscovered virus and others explain it by the existence of some intrinsic fault in the body. But even if we exclude these doubtful cases, it can safely be said that the majority of illnesses from which mankind suffers are directly, or indirectly, the result of microbial infection. It may well be that a clue to the meaning of disease will be found in an understanding of the function of micro-organisms in organic life.

When we looked at disease from the standpoint of the individual, we were unable to find any meaning in it, and were forced to regard it merely as an unfortunate accident. Now that we have stood further away from our subject, and have viewed illness on the larger scale of life on the earth, it begins to acquire a new significance. A disease caused by a pathogenic organism, instead of being a meaningless accident, is seen to be an inevitable consequence of the conditions obtaining in organic life on the earth. As we have seen, the components of this Great Life live on and through each other, a certain balance being maintained between them. From the point of view of humanity, an epidemic of influenza, such as that which swept through the world in 1918, was a disaster, but from the point of view of the virus which caused it, it was a triumph. During that year there was a temporary shifting of the balance in favour of certain pathogenic organisms, a shifting which was only corrected when mankind had mobilized its forces of resistance and overcome its enemy. Even in the absence of such serious epidemics as this, the scales are continually swinging backwards and forwards, each fluctuation in favour of the micro-organisms being followed by the re-establishment of a new balance. Painfully, but surely, the *status quo* is restored, only to be disturbed again by the attack of some new foe which catches us at a disadvantage. When we have got the measure of an enemy, our bodies manage to adopt the methods that are necessary for our defence. Should, however, a new and unfamiliar foe appear, we do not always know how to deal with it. This was well illustrated by the epidemic of measles which broke out amongst the Redskins of America during the last century. Never having encountered this disease before, and having no immunity to it, thousands of Red Indians succumbed to an illness which was a minor trouble to the great majority of contemporary Europeans. An epidemic may then be regarded as being a disturbance in the balance maintained between man and pathogenic organisms and may be caused either by an increase in the virulence of organisms, or else by a diminution in the resistance which man offers to them. Because under-nourishment, fatigue and poor conditions of life lead to a lowering of resistance, epidemics and pestilence are a frequent aftermath of war. At this very moment conditions are being created in Europe for a vast epidemic which in the end may cause more deaths than the war. Starvation, insanitary conditions of life, despair and fear, are sapping the resistance of the inhabitants of the occupied countries, and preparing the way for a violent disturbance of the balance maintained between mankind and the pathogenic micro-organisms.

Life feeds on life. Animals live on plants and in turn are eaten by animals more powerful than themselves, a certain mean being maintained between the eaters and the eaten. If there is a temporary upset of this balance in a particular locality, it is soon restored; a large number of some species of caterpillar appears in one part of this country and within a few days flocks of the very birds which feed on these caterpillars arrive to deal with the new pest. W. Aspden describes how when voles increased in a part of Scotland, short-eared owls flew from Scandinavia to restore the balance. By what means were the birds brought to the caterpillar-infested neighbourhood, and what prompted the owls to emigrate at that particular moment from Norway? Students of the science of ecology attempt to answer these questions, but it must be confessed that we know as little about the factors which regulate the balance between species as we do about those which control the growth of the various cells of the body.

Man, like all other forms of life on the earth, eats life, and in turn is eaten, not by those bigger and stronger than himself, but by those which are infinitely smaller and weaker. He is the prey of organisms which have adopted the parasitic mode of life, but this method of living is essentially the same as that employed by the carnivorae. Parasitism is only an expedient which a feeble organism·adopts in order to obtain food from the tissues of an organism which is too strong for it to be attacked by any other method. What the tiger is to the jungle deer, pathogenic organisms are to man; the tiger and the organisms are the eaters and jungle deer and man the eaten. The oscillations produced by epidemics are merely an example of the general biological principle that a truly stable equilibrium is never attained between the various species of life. Only when we examine the balance in the great aggregate of living creatures over long periods of time can the word equilibrium be used with any real justification.

The world of bacteria, moulds, plasmodia, and the world of the myriad unicellular inhabitants of the ocean, are of immense scientific and philosophical interest. It is a community of living creatures which is as ancient as it is ubiquitous. Bacteria are so old that they have been found in carboniferous and Devonian deposits, and there are many who believe that some simple organisms resembling bacteria or protozoa were the remote ancestors of all the varied life on this earth. This primitive world of micro-organisms occupies a kind of no-man's-land which lies midway between the vegetable and the animal kingdoms. They partake of the character of each. Some of them, such as the slime mould, creeps slowly over the surface of a rotting log like a gigantic amoeba and resembles an animal. Others, for example, the bacteria, are more closely allied to plants. Yet even amongst the bacteria there exists an immense diversity of form and function. Bacteria have been found which do not conform to a plant's method of living, resembling plants in their ability to build up simple into complex bodies, but differing from them in the fact that they are able to do this without the help of sunlight. The diversity of the world of micro-organisms, their variability and their plasticity is such as to fit them admirably for their rôle of filling the spaces lying between the animal and the vegetable kingdoms. If the various components of the great aggregate of life on the earth be compared with the different cells of the human body, then micro-organisms must be looked upon as being the connective tissue of the Great Life.

Bacteria reproduce themselves with such rapidity that a single bacterium, dividing every hour, may in the course of a day produce millions of millions of descendants, any one of which may display some slight variation from the orginal type. In order that animals and plants should exist, it would almost seem necessary that some simple and versatile form of life should be created to fill the gaps in the general pattern of life, and to make use of the various by-products of the vegetable and animal kingdoms. Bacteria fulfil both of these purposes admirably. By their diversity of form and function, the Life which covers the surface of the earth and penetrates into its outer layers is converted into a balanced and self-subsistent whole. If we make use of a geometrical figure as an illustration, it may be said that micro-organisms form, as it were, the base of a living triangle, the two sides of which are the vegetable and animal worlds. As this base approaches its junction with either side, it partakes more and more of the nature of that side, thus linking together the plants and the animals and completing the triangle of life.

Microbial disease may be looked upon as being one of the forms in which man makes payment to the great organism in which he lives, others being the sustenance he gives to the bacteria within him, the excreta he returns to the soil, and his body after his death. In the previous chapter illness was described as a state of inner disharmony which resulted from the combined action of strain and the impact of some external force. But there is no incompatibility between the various conclusions at which we have arrived. In illness there will often be discovered three components, the impact of hostile germs, the 'fifth column' action of strain and the defensive reaction on the part of the organism.

When Leeuwenhoek, the Delft draper and maker of the first microscope, peered at a drop of pond water and found that it was teeming with tiny living creatures, he did not realize the full import of his discovery. But those who received the news of Delft's discovery of minute living creatures were as thoroughly disquieted as were those who first learnt that the earth was not, as had hitherto been supposed, the centre and pivot of the universe. They felt that this profusion of minute organisms on the face of the globe detracted from the dignity of life and lowered the prestige of mankind. And if man were nothing but a living organism, they had reason to be perturbed. But man is more than this; he is mind and spirit, as well as body, in Nietzsche's compelling words, 'a hybrid of plant and ghost'. *Ex nihilo nihil.* Man's physical being is only a unit in the total film of life covering the surface of the earth. May not his spirit also be part of a greater spirit, his consciousness part of a greater consciousness? Nothing exists alone; everything forms part of a great whole. Forms and divisions are but the product of man's limited perception and mode of thought.

CHAPTER III

THE MISUSE OF FEAR

MAN's situation, like that of all other components of life on the earth, is, as we have seen, a precarious one. However cleverly he may scheme, whatever the dispositions his brain may allow him to make, he cannot escape from the laws controlling that great aggregate of life in which he finds himself. In his arrogance he may boast that he is conquering nature, but nature does not even fight; she is secure in her possession of his body. He may think that with a little more contriving he will be able to live out the span of his life, not only with security, but with reasonable comfort. This is an illusion, for there can be no security and no certainty of comfort for anything that breathes and moves.

The artificial conditions which civilized man has created for himself have done much to encourage this false belief that he is acquiring power over nature. By a touch of the finger the darkness around him is flooded with artificial sunlight; pressing a button he can be conveyed to the top of the house without moving a limb. He would seem to have banished the austerities of nature from his cities. As a result he tends to look upon security and comfort as being his by inalienable right. Carlyle inveighs with characteristic fervour against the fictitious standards which civilized man has created for himself:

> By certain valuations, and averages, of our own striking, we come upon some sort of average terrestrial lot; this we fancy belongs to us by nature, and of indefeasible right. It is simple payment of our wages, of our deserts; requires neither thanks nor complaint; only such *overplus* as there may be do we account Happiness; any *deficit* again is Misery. Now consider that we have the valuation of our own deserts ourselves, and what a fund of Self-conceit there is in each of us, — do you wonder that the balance should so often dip the wrong way, and many a Blockhead cry See there, what a payment; was ever worthy gentleman so used? — I tell thee, Blockhead, it all comes of thy Vanity; of what thou *fanciest* those same deserts of thine to be. Fancy that thou deservest

C

to be hanged (as is most likely), thou wilt feel it happiness to be only ˙shot: fancy that thou deservest to be hanged in a hair-halter, it will be a luxury to die in hemp (*Sartor Resartus.*)

Whilst it may not be necessary for us to lower our expectations to the nadir of a hair-halter, some lowering is necessary. For the body and the senses there can be no safety, and we must accept this as our human lot. Into these conditions of life we have been born, and for them we have been specially equipped. We have been thrown into the mêlée of life without any guarantee having been given for our safety. But, like our humbler partners in organic life, we have been provided with certain contrivances which warn us of the presence of danger and help us to escape from it. We have been equipped for a journey which of necessity must be perilous and we must not delude ourselves that it can ever be otherwise. Having discussed the conditions under which we live and the nature of disease, we can now turn from the general to the particular. In other words, we can leave for the moment large-scale phenomena and return to the more familiar happenings of the consulting-room.

If a statistically-minded physician were to go through his notes and tabulate the various symptoms of which his patients complained, and were then to place these in order of frequency, he would find that the commonest ill from which his patients suffered was fear. Having discovered this he might proceed to classify the types of fear which were responsible for his patients coming to consult him. He would find that sometimes the fear was the cause, and sometimes the result of their illness. Sometimes the patient was aware of it, and sometimes entirely unconscious of the explanation of his suffering. Sometimes the fear revealed itself in the preliminary remarks with which the patient opened the conversation, and sometimes it only became obvious as he was about to leave. The following may be regarded as being a fair sample of those significant parting words which often disclose the existence of fear.

'Then you don't think, doctor, that there is anything seriously wrong with me?'

'No. What were you frightened of?'

'I don't know — something really serious.'

Fears grow best in darkness, and should be dragged into the daylight.

When a patient is too frightened to name what he fears, firm treatment is necessary, as in the handling of nettles. The accursed thing must be grasped boldly and uprooted. 'What actually did you think you might be suffering from?'

'Oh, some sort of growth.' Still the patient evades the fearsome name, indicating that further help is required.

'You mean cancer?' There is a sudden tightening of the muscles of the patient's face, a momentary pause, and then admission, often conveyed only by a movement of the head. The horrid thing has been dragged to the surface, and being clearly visible, can be dispatched. The exposure of a fear and its subsequent destruction may be all that is required to restore the inner harmony known as health.

But terror of that highly dramatized malady, cancer, is not the only cause of the anxious expression so often seen in the consulting-room. There is the fear of the patient who believes that an operation will be necessary, and the fear of the man who is struggling to support his wife and family, and who knows that a long illness will entail suffering not only for himself, but for them. There is the fear of the financially-minded man who looks on everything in terms of money, and who has calculated in a flash the expenses of the nursing home and operation. There is the less well-defined fear of the patient who has hitherto accepted life as a secure possession and who is suddenly made to realize that it may be only a loan. This is more likely to attack the hale and the strong, who, because they have never come face to face with illness, have dwelt in the comforting illusion that whatever may befall their friends they themselves are immune to disaster. Finally, there is the fear of pain, of growing old, of suffering and death, fears that seem so natural that some people regard them as being physiological. It is only when these fears are out of all proportion to any suffering which an illness is likely to entail that special attention must be directed to them. A doctor must always be on the alert, for fear does not always look out from the patient's eyes. Sometimes it is covered by a studied non-chalance, uncalled-for laughter or braggadocio. There is even the most subtly disguised of all, the fear of showing fear, the fear which has earned so many decorations on the battlefield.

Because fear is universal and is the cause of so much suffering, it will be helpful to study it in greater detail, and more particularly, its mechanism. This study is facilitated by the fact that fear is one of the great primitive emotions common to men and animals, a mechanism which has been given to them for their safety. Because it is physiological as well as pathological, fear can be brought within the range of experimental methods of investigation. By means of laboratory experiments we can study not only its external manifestations, but also its paths within the body, from its outposts in the sense organs to its headquarters in the brain. But before describing its physiology a few words must be said concerning the psychological aspects of fear. Like other emotions fear is not simply a certain quality of experience, but an experience to which is attached a conative element, or factor of effort. When we are afraid we become conscious of a striving within us, of a reaction of the body associated with the emotional feeling: we are aware, not only of painful impressions, but of a compelling urge to escape or to defend ourselves. Both of these components, the painful impression and the reaction, enter into the emotion of fear, and together constitute the mechanism which secures our escape from danger.

It is important to note that, whilst processes of thought seem to be localized in the head, emotions are felt throughout the whole of the body. When a man suddenly comes face to face with danger, vibrations of fear run through his physical being; he experiences a sinking in the pit of the stomach, he breaks out in a cold sweat, his skin becomes pale, his mouth dry, his breathing difficult and his heart races. His sensations are as widespread as is the network of nerves along which its messages run; he is frightened throughout the whole expanse of his body. To understand why this is so we must have an elementary knowledge of the anatomy and physiology of the central nervous system. This consists of the brain, its prolongation (the spinal cord), and the numerous nerves which arise from these two structures. In all popular works on physiology the central nervous system is likened to a network of telegraph wires, which keeps the headquarters of the brain in touch with the events taking place in the rest of the body. The function of the central nervous system is to co-ordinate the manifold activities of the body and to maintain its contact with the outside world. Some nerves, such as those responsible for the movement of the limbs, are under the control of the will, and are termed voluntary, whilst others, regulating inner functions, are automatic, and collectively are known as the autonomic, or sympathetic system. The autonomic system consists of a fine network of nerve-fibres spread throughout the body, which in certain situations becomes denser, to form what are known as ganglia and plexuses. The best known of these local collections of nerve-fibres is the solar plexus, which lies in the upper part of the abdomen, and which, to older systems of medicine, was the centre of the emotional life. The solar plexus is an important part of the sympathetic system, and, since the whole of this system is intimately connected with emotional experiences, the old idea that this structure was the seat of the emotions is not without justification. But whilst the modern physiologist would frankly admit the importance of the solar plexus, he would locate the centre of the emotional life in two large masses of grey matter which lie at the base of the brain. These nuclei, known as the thalami, are particularly well developed in the lower animals, and it is in them that the fibres of the sympathetic system finally lose themselves. In man the thalami are less conspicuous because they are swamped by the great cerebral hemispheres, which are the seat of his intellectual activity. Important fibres connect the more instinctive parts of the brain (the thalami) with the front areas of the cerebral hemispheres (the organ of man's higher faculties). Here, in the part of the brain which lies behind the brow, thoughts receive their emotional tone from the impulses conveyed to them from the thalami. Not only do the thalami influence the cerebral hemispheres, but the cerebral hemispheres influence the thalami, intellect and feeling continually reacting upon each other. If, when walking down a road at night, we see a dark mass in our path, the more primitive parts of our brain come into action, and we experience an instantaneous spasm of fear. A moment later we realize that the menacing dark shape is only a bush, and the fear disappears. By explaining to us the true nature of the threatening shadow the cerebral hemispheres have put a brake on the activity of the thalamus. The moderating action of the cerebral hemispheres on the subjacent structures can be demonstrated by animal experiments. It is possible to remove the whole of an animal's cerebral hemispheres without causing death. When a cat is subjected to this mutilation, it remains in a state of perpetual rage and fear. The slightest movement in its vicinity throws it into a frenzy of fear and anger; it bares its teeth, erects the hairs on its back and spits.

It is entirely controlled by the thalamic or more automatic levels of its brain.

This observation is of great importance to our understanding of the mechanics of fear in human beings, and explains one of the subjects dealt with in the previous chapter. We saw there that certain illnesses, such as asthma, are the result of an overaction of the body, and that similar examples could be found of overaction of the mind. There are patients who remain in a perpetual state of alarm, and who react so violently to hostile forces that the mildest stimulation produces profound disturbances. It is not their reaction which is abnormal, but its exaggerated nature. Generally this lack of balance is due to a failure on the part of the cerebral hemispheres to exercise a moderating action on the thalamus.

Fear causes many physiological changes in the body in addition to the more obvious manifestations already enumerated. When we are frightened a large amount of sugar is excreted into the blood, and the adrenal glands (aptly termed the glands of emergency) suddenly become intensely active, pouring their secretions into the veins. To compensate for this increased activity of certain organs during a fear crisis there is a temporary suspension of the non-essential functions of the body, such as digestion, all the energies of the body being concentrated on the task of escaping from danger. According to the James-Lange theory, these bodily manifestations of fear are not the *result* of the emotion, but the *cause* of it. As William James put it:

> ... the more rational statement is that we feel sorry because we cry, angry because we strike, afraid because we tremble, and not that we cry, strike or tremble, because we are sorry, angry or fearful, as the case may be. Without the bodily states following on the perception, the latter would be purely cognitive in form, pale, colourless, destitute of emotional warmth.

James went on to say:

> Emotion dissociated from all bodily feelings is inconceivable. The more closely I scrutinize my states, the more persuaded I become that whatever moods, affections and passions I have, are, in very truth, constituted by, and made up of, those body changes which we ordinarily call their expression and consequence.

The back-flow of impressions which, in James's view, impart richness of feeling to the emotions, comes, as has already been emphasized, from all parts of the body, from the muscles, the blood vessels, the skin and the viscera. James gives to the viscera an important rôle in the genesis of the emotions, thereby reminding us of the Old Testament sayings, 'his bowels yearned', and 'his bowels were turned to water'. But the majority of physiologists do not accept the 'James-Lange' theory of the emotions, and Sherrington claims to have disproved it by experiments on animals. He divided the spinal cord of a dog so as to abolish all messages reaching the brain from the viscera, and found that the animal still displayed the emotional behaviour typical of joy, anger or disgust. But these experiments are inconclusive, for whatever its behaviour may have been, it was not possible for Sherrington to have known whether the dog actually *felt* the emotions appropriate to its actions. We need not concern ourselves with the correctness or incorrectness of the James-Lange theory. All that is of importance is that we should realize that the whole of the body is pervaded by the emotion of fear, and that few structures in it escape its influence.

Fear is purposive and useful, a fact which Darwin long ago recognized when he described it as being a 'serviceable associated action'. Its function is to mobilize as quickly as possible all the resources of the body, either for combat or for escape. Most emotions lead to action, but in the great majority of cases the conative, or striving element is less urgent, and action need not be taken immediately. But fear brooks no delay, and in an instant the whole body must be ready for flight or combat. When the fear reaction of an animal is excessive, it may defeat its own purpose, the animal remaining immobilized in terror. Also if fear persists, it can no longer act as an alarm notifying the presence of some new danger. It is amongst human beings that we find the most striking examples of the mechanism of fear being misused; through the stimulus of the imagination it is brought into action unnecessarily or else persists when danger no longer threatens. Amongst animals fear is more likely to function normally. When a creature of the wood senses danger, its body reacts, and then, when the danger has passed, resumes its normal state; it does not remain immobilized in a state of perpetual anxiety. Julian Duguid, in an excellent description of life in South American forests, points out that it is an error to believe that the jungle is the home of ceaseless terror. Even although its inhabitants walk in danger of their lives, their reactions of fear are but short lived; the startled deer bounds a few hundred yards into safety and then resumes its nibbling, oblivious of the danger which a few moments before had galvanized it into action; the monkeys scurrying in panic across the treetops soon settle again to their fascinating search for vermin in each other's pelts; the crocodile, disturbed out of its coma, resumes its lethargy almost before its body has reached the refuge of the water. If it were otherwise, life in the jungle would be wellnigh impossible. Not only would the bodies of the jungle inhabitants be worn out by the continuous strain imposed upon them, but they would have the greatest difficulty in obtaining the necessary nourishment for the continuation of life. Because digestion is suspended during fear an animal which remained perpetually mobilized would die in the end of inanition.

Civilized man, by the cunning of his hand and by his wonder-working cerebral cortex, has succeeded in escaping from the primitive life of the jungle, and, in times of peace, has won for himself some degree of security from physical perils. He no longer walks in perpetual danger of violence and sudden death; but, alas, he has only exchanged one form of insecurity for another. The physical jungle has disappeared, but we still walk in the dim jungle created by our imagination, a make-believe wilderness full of intangible horrors. Because their anxiety seldom reaches the level of terror, and because the bodily changes which are associated with it are likely to pass unnoticed, few people realize how big a place fear occupies in their lives. A patient may boast that he is entirely free from worry, and yet be living a life of low-grade anxiety. What renders the condition of such a man deplorable is that his anxieties, unlike those evoked by the jungle, are of his own contriving. He is worrying about what will never happen, but unfortunately, the results are as devastating as though it had happened. A train of thought starts in a man's cerebral cortex, and an imaginary situation is reviewed. 'Suppose that attack of indigestion which I had last Tuesday turned out to be an early symptom of cancer?' 'Perhaps my shares will fall instead of rising . . .' 'If the train's late again I may miss my appointment.' Beaconsfield wrote, 'There is always something to worry you. It comes as regularly as sunrise', and

Beaconsfield was an acute observer. There is no event of daily life too trivial to be surrounded with an aura of worry. One may make onself miserable over the possibility that the toast may be burnt again at breakfast, the corner seat in the carriage taken, or the likelihood that the office typist will have one of her irritating fidgety moods again. This is the quality of the emotions which make up our inner life. These may be the daylong thoughts and feelings of the patient who has boasted that he hasn't a care in the world. Only the indefinable expression of the eyes, the slight tightening of the muscles of the face advertise to the acute observer that he is never really at ease, never relaxed. He walks in a jungle of petty self-created fears. His cerebral cortex is for ever whispering of imaginary dangers to the centres at the base of the brain. As a result muscles are kept tightened, adrenalin is poured into his blood-stream, and a muted panic pervades his whole body.

How easily imaginary pictures formed in the cerebral cortex may conjure up fear is shown by a simple experiment. If a plank is laid on the ground none of us will have any difficulty in walking along it. But place it across a stream and for many of us the plank becomes a tight-rope. Imagination now works at high speed and we see ourselves falling headlong into the stream. Warnings are shouted into the thalamus and fear takes possession of us. We dare not walk across that plank.

What distinguishes most of our fear reactions from those of the animals is that instead of being serviceable, they are harmful, since they are provoked by a danger that exists only in our imagination. Such fears but rarely lead to the taking of any appropriate action. When we are alarmed and angered by the motorist who drives in the middle of the road in front of us, we may wish to murder him, but we take no steps to do so. He remains unscathed whilst we, his would-be assailants, are hit by our own boomerang of anger. Our inner processes have been speeded up, adrenalin has been poured into the blood-stream, and at the same time a strong brake has been applied to all action. Inner friction has been raised to a maximum and nothing has been achieved. It may be objected that misuse of the fear mechanism is not confined to human beings, and that a rabbit, instead of being mobilized for flight, may remain immobilized by terror. As in the case of the enraged motorist the body has been prepared for action and no action has been taken. This is undoubtedly true. The immobility of the rabbit is another example of a purposeful action overreaching itself, and thus defeating its aim. Similar instances were given in Chapter 1, where certain illnesses, such as asthma, were described which were found to be due to overaction of the organism to a stimulus. Other examples of a disproportionate response to a stimulus will be given later when we come to deal with the subject of pain. All these examples of ill-balanced action indicate that the idea that perfection is necessarily an attribute of nature must be abandoned. Nature, like man, is subject to error. Sometimes she overshoots her mark, and her mechanisms defeat the very purpose for which they were created. But because a rabbit is sometimes immobilized by terror, instead of being galvanized into action, there is no need for us to question the purposive nature of fear. Because an anxious mother has given extra milk to her child under the impression that it is under-nourished, and has thereby provoked a bilious attack, we do not doubt the nutritive value of milk. Nor need we question the purposive action of fear, because in excess, it defeats its own ends.

Weighed down by anxiety and constantly mobilized for action, it is small wonder that modern civilized man suffers from nervous troubles, gastric disturbances and vascular ailments. Because anxiety is so widespread that it is the rule rather than the exception, it has come to be regarded as the normal lot of man. To such an extent do people accept worry as right and proper, that they are even disturbed when a man is not sufficiently upset by the alarums and excursions of life. Occasionally this attitude is justified, for there are people whose equanimity is based, not on a philosophical attitude to life, but on indifferences and callousness to all that does not touch their own personal comfort and convenience.

There is no panacea for the strain of modern life short of the achievement of sainthood, for only saints and the great sages have succeeded in conquering fear and in living without taking thought for the morrow. Few people can become saints, but even an ordinary man can eliminate a great deal of fear if he attains a workable philosophy of life. It is because of the absence of any positive beliefs and because we seem to be alone in a vast impersonal universe dependent for survival on our own efforts that we are so troubled. A little science has gone to our heads, and the power of religion has declined.

This I dare affirm in knowledge of nature [wrote Francis Bacon], that a little natural philosophy, and the first entrance into it, doth dispose the opinion to atheism; but on the other side, much natural philosophy, and wading deep into it, will bring about men's minds to religion. (*Meditationes Sacrae.*)

We men and women of the present day are at the stage of 'a little natural philosophy'. We have analysed the body, and because we have done this some of us have imagined that the mystery of life has been eliminated. We have measured the sun, and because we have discovered that it is only a star of the second magnitude we no longer wonder at its mysterious splendour. God has become an unnecessary hypothesis to the possessor of 'a little natural philosophy'. And now the 'enlightenment' of the West is spreading Eastward and the bowler-hatted Mohammedan of to-day finds it difficult to bow his head and murmur, as did his fathers, 'It is the Will of Allah'.

When a patient is totally unaware of the nature of the fear which troubles him, and when it is not obvious to his physician, he may sometimes be helped by analytical treatment. If he can become aware of that which troubles him, he may be able to find a new attitude to it. In order that he may attain peace his cerebral cortex must cease to talk frighteningly to his already alarmed thalamus, and his critical faculties must be brought to bear on the extravagant creations of his imagination. As a beginning he should be encouraged to examine the blackest products of his mind. What is the worst that could possibly befall him? When the particular bogy which frightens him has been dragged into the daylight, and thoroughly surveyed, it will often be found to be nothing more substantial than a sheet and a broomstick. The imagination is a brilliant writer of tragedies, but of tragedies which are convincing only when played in a dim light. If the illumination be increased, their burlesque nature immediately becomes apparent. Towards the end of his life Mark Twain wrote: 'I am an old man, and I have had a great many troubles; and most of them have never happened.' It is a comment which most elderly people could make.

CHAPTER IV

PAIN

MEREDITH wrote: 'There is purpose in pain; otherwise it were devilish.' He was right in his surmise. Pain has much in common with fear, and like it, is an instrument for the apprehension of danger. But when pain sounds the alarm the danger has already reached the body. It utters a sharp and unmistakable warning that the organism is being injured, and that it is necessary to escape. Or, if the damage which has already been done is sufficiently serious — as in the case of a sprained ankle — pain enforces rest of the injured part in order that it may recover. Even the simplest animal automatically shuns discomfort, and, without question, moves in the direction of comfort. A child who has put his finger too near to the fascinating flame, withdraws it with a speed that exceeds the quickness of thought. An alarm signal has been flashed along the pain nerves running from the hand to the brain, and urgent return messages have been sent out to the muscles of the arm. This pain reflex is obviously an automatic safety mechanism, which preserves the child's hand from damage. We have only to see what happens when pain reflexes are abolished to realize that they are given to us for our benefit and not for our annoyance. A patient who suffers from that strange and rare disease of the central nervous system, syringomyelia, retains his sense of touch but cannot appreciate heat, cold, or pain. As a result he is unconscious of discomfort when his hand is in contact with a flame or a sharp point, and damages himself so frequently that one or more fingers have often to be amputated. He is a living testimonial to the value of pain.

But as happens with other devices of nature the mechanism of pain does not always work satisfactorily. Pain, like fear or like the reaction of certain organs to stimuli, is sometimes so excessive, or so prolonged, as to defeat its own purpose. Instead of ensuring the immobilization of the enflamed, or damaged, structure, pain may be so exaggerated as to lead to a disturbance of the whole organism. This overreaching of the mark is frequently seen in medical practice. A pain response is sometimes so overwhelming that it is only after the doctor has reduced it by the use of morphia that the patient is able to rest. It is not without reason that opium is sometimes referred to as 'the gift of the gods' These cases of excessive pain are another instance of an exaggerated response defeating the aim for which it was initiated. In the physical and in the spiritual world alike it is the 'Middle Way' that leads to salvation.

Pain sensations arise in special nerve endings scattered over the surface of the body which differ from those of touch and temperature by being naked or without specialized coverings. From the surfaces of the body pain impulses are conducted along special tracts in the spinal cord to arrive eventually at the same destination as that reached by fear impulses, namely, the thalami at the base of the brain. The similarity between the anatomy and physiology of pain and of fear does not end here. Pain sensations in the thalamus, like those of fear, are relayed by association fibres to the sensory areas of the cerebral cortex, where they become more conscious. And just as this higher part of the brain exercises a certain degree of control over fear messages, so can it decide within limits how the organism will react to pain. When pain is sharp and unexpected, it provokes flight, a loud cry, a leap to one side, or resistance to the hostile agent which is responsible for the injury. This is an automatic action, and an example of primitive, instinctive behaviour, uncontrolled by the cerebral cortex. Should the pain messages be less insistent the cerebral cortex may merely register them and decline all action. If at the same time a multitude of highly exciting messages of another nature are reaching the cortex, and its attention is thus fully occupied, the pain may not even become conscious. This failure to respond to pain is seen in hysterical patients and in those who are under the influence of great excitement. A soldier advancing on the battlefield may not even know that he is wounded until he sees the bloodstains on his tunic.

Langdon Brown points out that although pain sensations are less easily provoked than are those coming from the special sense organs, when they have been aroused they are explosive in character. Another of their characteristics is that they tend to persist even after the stimulus which produced them has been removed. Langdon Brown illustrates these two points by means of the experiment of plunging the hand into water of different temperatures.

At the right temperature water will give merely a pleasant sensation of warmth, but if you put your hand in water that is just too hot, the painful sensation comes perceptibly later than that of warmth. You may be able to bear the immersion of the hand, but if you increase the stimulated area by plunging in the whole arm, the number of painful impressions will mount up unbearably. Moreover, the pain will persist after you have withdrawn your arm because, as Sir Thomas Lewis has shown, a chemical substance exciting pain has been set free. (SIR WALTER LANGDON BROWN: *Thus we are Men*.)

This simple experiment illustrates three characteristics of pain: its explosive nature, its persistence after the stimulus has ceased, and the fact that its intensity depends on the number of pain fibres which have been stimulated.

When we analyse any painful experience we find that it can be resolved into two components: an unpleasant sensation and an emotional reaction to this. The relative importance of these two elements in pain varies with different people and on different occasions. Sometimes the emotional reaction is so intense as to be quite out of proportion to the sensation. An exaggerated emotional response is seen in tired and distressed patients whose resistance has been worn down by suffering. There is a point at which the morale of each of us suddenly snaps; there is a limit to what we can bear. I am not referring here to a physiological limit, but to the psychic capacity to endure. It frequently happens that after an operation followed by a trying convalescence, a patient's powers of resistance suddenly fail. Up till that moment he willingly submitted to treatment, but he is now thrown into a state of intense apprehension at the thought of any further discomfort, even although this be negligible compared with what he has previously borne. From being an easily handled patient he becomes one who is quite incapable of co-operating with his nurses and doctors. He is supersensitive, like the princess in the fairy-tale who could detect the presence of a pea beneath seven layers of feather mattresses. He has become allergic like a man who after receiving a series of injections of serum suddenly develops an intense antipathy to it.

The question of different thresholds of pain, in other words, of

46

varying degrees of sensitiveness, is of the greatest interest to medical men. Clinical experience shows that few people react identically to the same painful stimulus; what provokes only discomfort in one patient apparently causes acute agony to another. There are two possible explanations of this variability: the first a difference in the sensibility of the nerves conveying the message of pain, the second a difference in the control exercised over the thalamus by the cerebral cortex. In the example of the patient broken down by suffering the explanation is undoubtedly a weakening of cortical control. The tired cerebral cortex no longer attempts to hold in check the automatic responses of the lower levels of the brain. It may even increase these responses by the whisperings of an extravagant imagination. 'I can bear no more', 'I have come to an end', 'They're going to hurt me again', 'I am afraid and would sooner die'. Instead of exercising a moderating influence the cerebral cortex rings alarm bells in the thalamus and maintains it in a continuous state of panic.

In striking contrast to the tired patient is the patient who suffers pain with a minimum of emotional reaction to it. Such a patient is conscious of unpleasant sensations, but has no anxiety or fear concerning them. The pain is a warning that something is wrong with the body and that appropriate remedial measures must be adopted. If nothing can be done to bring immediate relief the philosophically-minded patient directs his attention, so far as is possible, in other directions. Even before the physiology of pain was understood Seneca realized that this was the best method of combating it. 'The more the attention is fixed on the cause which produces pain, the more its intensity is increased, the more a man stands away from it, the more relief he gets.' Pascal once demonstrated the truth of Seneca's saying in a way that few people could imitate. He suffered from severe 'tic douloureux' (facial neuralgia), and one night this became so insistent that he gave up all hope of sleep. In order to divert his mind from his physical misery he determined to concentrate his thoughts on the problem of the Cycloid, which had long been the despair of geometricians, and solved it during the night. His patron, the Duke de Roannes, who was also a mathematician, was very much excited by the news, and asked what use he intended to make of this discovery: 'None', answered Pascal, it was but the cure for a bad night.' Although few have such control over their attention as had Pascal, there are great differences in the extent to which patients are subjugated by their pains. Two men may suffer from the same condition — for example, an incurable cancer of the tongue. One of them admits that he suffers pain, but spurning self-pity, he continues to work as long as he can, and endeavours to maintain his interest in everything which has previously enriched his life. The other gives up all his activities, retires to bed, and devotes his whole time to noting the variations in his discomfort. He is full of self-pity and is prostrated by his pain. But, as has already been said, there is a limit to the amount of physical suffering which can be endured, and it is the point at which this limit is reached which varies so widely in different people. What applies to pain applies also to illness. Seneca might have said with equal truth: 'The more the attention is fixed on illness, the more its intensity is increased; the more a man can stand away from it, the more relief he is likely to get.' If, when ill, one can contrive not to be completely lost in the body, if one can feel some existence apart from it, the effect of the illness will be lessened.

One of the obstacles to a scientific study of pain is that it is a purely subjective phenomenon. We have no means of measuring its intensity. But little reliance can be placed on words, for as a rule the more extravagant the terms in which a patient describes his sensations, the less intense is his pain likely to be. Those who are really in agony speak very little, for they have great difficulty in making the physical and mental efforts necessary for speech. Not by any words that they may utter, but by their pallor, their tense muscles, their dilated pupils, and by the cold sweat on their brow, does one realize the extent of their suffering. Attempts have been made to find a rough test of pain sensibility in different people. The test most commonly used is to press the thumb against a bony outgrowth which may be felt at the junction of the neck and the skull, and which is known as the styloid process. By employing this test patients have been graded into three classes according to the amount of pressure required to elicit a pain response, the hypo-sensitive (under-sensitive), the sensitive and the hyper-sensitive (over-sensitive). The first group includes those who, when the test is applied, neither complain nor give evidence of experiencing pain. In the second group are those who, on being questioned, admit that they felt discomfort, and in the third group are those who react strongly, and complain bitterly. The test is lacking in accuracy, but yields interesting information. Those who have used it state that the reaction to pain varies greatly in different individuals, and in the same person under different conditions. Anxiety, insomnia, fatigue and illness, all tend to increase a man's sensibility to pain by weakening the control exercised over it by the cerebral cortex. Good health, rest and excitement have an opposite effect. The influence of excitement on pain has already been noted. Occupation would also appear to have some influence on sensibility to pain. Libman found that 90 per cent of the professional boxers whom he tested in New York were hypo-sensitive. He also reported that 98 per cent of full-blooded Red Indians had an abnormally high threshold to pain, in other words, they were comparatively insensitive to it. This not only bears out the popular view of the Redskin but also to some extent supports Ribot's view that sensibility to pain is proportional to a nation's level of civilization. If Ribot be right, we pay for our culture by a capacity to suffer, a view which was held by Lombroso. This writer stated that habitual criminals, and more especially those imprisoned for acts of violence, showed marked indifference to their own sufferings. Research at the Cornell Medical College in New York suggests that the capacity to endure pain does not depend so much on variations in the sensitiveness of the pain nerve-fibres, as on the control exercised over the thalamus by the cerebral hemispheres. The pain threshold of different people was measured by focusing heat rays from an electric lamp on to the forehead and noting the amount of heat required to produce a sensation of pain. This proved to be more or less the same for everybody, namely, 0.21 gram calories per second per square centimetre of skin exposed to light.

The body is equipped with a number of different safety devices which regulate its functions somewhat as the 'governors' of an engine control its speed. When a reaction becomes too violent, these braking mechanisms are set going. The capacity to feel pain is subject to such control. When a certain intensity of pain has been reached no more can be felt, even although the stimulus be doubled, owing to the patient having lost consciousness. The intense pain has produced a reflex inhibition of the heart which diminishes the circulation through the brain and causes the patient to faint. It must be remembered that the brain is more sensitive than any other tissue in the body to changes in its environment. For example, Haldane has calculated that an increase of about one in twenty thousand million parts in the proportion by weight of ionized hydrogen present in the brain is sufficient to cause loss of consciousness. We have only to take three or four deep breaths of pure nitrogen or hydrogen in order to wash out from the lungs the oxygen they contain, and consciousness disappears. It is not surprising therefore that a severe disturbance in another part of the body is likely to cause loss of consciousness.

Thanks to this mechanism the ingenuity of torturers is finally thwarted, and their victims are saved from the refinements of agony which they have contrived. We can also derive some comfort from the thought that the spiritual exaltation in which the martyrs met their deaths probably exercised a strong influence over their sufferings. It is well known that many religious devotees, such as those belonging to the sect of Howling Dervishes, are able to endure pain which no ordinary man could tolerate.

Hitherto we have discussed only pain resulting from the peripheral, or surface, stimulation of the pain nerves. But just as it is possible to ring an electric bell by direct manipulation, and without touching the bell push, so can pain be evoked by a stimulus in the central structures of the brain. This centrally aroused pain is generally the result of emotional stresses. Conflicting desires, and destructive emotions such as constant irritation, prolonged resentment, anxiety and self-pity, are potent causes of illness which may be manifested either in the psyche as depression, mental fatigue, etc., or in the body as disturbance of function, or pain. It is important to realize that when a patient feels pain of central origin or what is known as psychogenic pain it is as real as that caused by the irritation of nerve endings; it must never be lightly dismissed on the grounds that it is imaginary. And just as peripherally aroused pain is a danger-signal that something is amiss with the body, so must centrally aroused pain be regarded as a warning that all is not well with the psyche. The sufferer from psychogenic pain is as much in need of help as is the patient who displays a lesion which is obviously responsible for his discomfort. Unfortunately the psychic causes of pain are not so apparent as are those of peripheral origin and the explanation of the trouble varies widely in different cases. Sometimes a patient feels pain because this provides him with the only available escape from an emotional dilemma. When a patient makes use of this centrally-engendered pain in order to escape from a situation which has proved too difficult for him, he is quite unaware of what he is doing. Neither the soldier who avails himself of pain as a means of avoiding battle, nor the worker who adopts the same ruse in order to leave a detested occupation, are guilty of fraud. In protesting that the last thing they want to do is to shirk their duty, and that if only they could get rid of their pain they would willingly carry on, they are quite sincere, for they are totally unaware of the conflict which is being waged in the depths of their mind, the conflict between the instinct of self-preservation and the acquired ideals of self-respect and duty.

It is difficult for a layman, and especially for a patient, to realize that real pain can be felt even although there be no physical cause for it. Attempts on the part of a doctor to explain the nature of psychogenic pain are usually interrupted. 'Then you think I am imagining this pain? Well, I'm not. It's very real.' This is the indignant reply which often follows the doctor's efforts to throw light on the nature of psychogenic pain. All that the doctor has succeeded in doing is to have provided his patient with two new grievances: first, that the doctor has minimized his difficulties; and second, that he has cast reflections on his character. Whilst nobody can be blamed for being ill, a stigma is attached to wrong working of the mind. This being so the sufferer from psychogenic pain feels, in the expressive words of the East, that he has lost 'face'.

This fear of losing 'face' is an important motive in human behaviour and pain is sometimes used as a means of 'saving face'. Let us take as an example a man with high ambitions and a desire for the world's respect who finds that he is unable to realize his dreams. Because he is unable to admit failure even to himself, much less to his friends, he develops a functional illness which forces him to retire from his work. This, he announces, is the explanation of his lack of success, and by this simple device he not only saves his 'face', but also gains the sympathy of his friends. No fraud has been perpetrated because he himself is convinced that but for his unfortunate illness he would have succeeded. Sometimes the intentional character of the pain is revealed by the fact that it is expressly suited to the purposes for which it is being used. A girl whose whole ambition is to become an artist and who has been forced to take up typewriting for a living may easily develop cramp in the hand. These cramps will entirely disappear if she is allowed to use her hand for painting.

The difficulty we experience in understanding how a psychological conflict can produce pain is partly due to our having accepted the Cartesian philosophy that mind and body are separate entities. And it is not only the neurotic patient but the philosopher also who finds difficulty in explaining how mind and body can interact. Numerous and ingenious solutions of this enigma have been offered, but they are all unsatisfactory. The Cartesian division into mind and body served a purpose in allowing man's body to be studied first, but it has now led to an impasse and must be abandoned. Instead of placing mind and body in two separate categories we must regard them as being different aspects of a single entity. If we adopt this new standpoint, we are compelled to abandon the former division of illnesses into functional and structural, psychic and somatic. Disturbances of function cause structural changes, and structural changes disturbances of function; emotional conflicts produce tension of muscles, overactivity of certain glands and changes in the circulation. Conversely these changes in the body give rise to emotional disturbances; fear causes adrenalin to be poured into the circulation, and if adrenalin be injected into a vein, a normal man is made to feel afraid; tense muscles lead to anxiety, and indigestion to irritability. The words functional and organic, psychic and somatic may still be used as convenient labels for indicating the centre of gravity of an illness, but they no longer express any difference of a fundamental nature.

A patient suffering from psychogenic pain frequently makes use of some trivial organic trouble which, had it not been for his emotional difficulties, would have been of little importance to him. There is a condition familiar to doctors which often follows a railway accident, and is consequently known as 'railway spine' The patient develops pain in the back, which may be irradiated along any of the nerves running out of the spinal cord. So long as negotiations with the railway company are in progress, all remedies fail to give relief, but immediately the compensation has been settled, the condition rapidly clears up. The mechanism of 'railway spine' can be easily understood. The accident caused some minor lesion, such as bruising and tearing of muscle fibres, which, but for the mental disturbance, would soon have ceased to cause pain. But the self-seeking, or self-pitying, submerged portion of the patient's mind avails itself of this lesion to further its own ends. When these have been served the pain disappears.

Pain may be used by the less conscious parts of the mind for a great many other purposes, amongst others for the attainment of power. However poor his natural endowments may be, a sick person establishes for himself a privileged position in the household. The querulous and domineering invalid is so well-known a figure as to have become a favourite theme for novelists and playwrights, and Molière's *Malade Imaginaire*, and Somerset Maugham's *The Mollusc*, are examples of works written around this subject. Again it must be stressed that these power-seeking and face-saving invalids are not usually aware of the truth. Nature has provided us with excellent blinkers, which, by restricting the field of our vision, enable us to avoid seeing whatever is displeasing. And the truth, and more especially the truth about ourselves, is not always agreeable; it is more likely to be stern and forbidding. Tiresome though these self-deceived men and women generally are, they are the victims of the unseen workings of their own minds, and are to be pitied rather than blamed. Sometimes they are vaguely aware of the turmoil within them, and of the discrepancy between their ideals and their attainments. This is not infrequently explained by the fact that these ideals are based on an utterly false conception of the world and of their own importance. What makes the lot of these people so difficult is that their capacity to endure is weakened by the inner dissension which is itself the cause of their illness. The enemy has established himself in what man has fondly described as 'the citadel of the mind'.

This theory of pain, namely, that it is a danger signal indicating the presence of physical or of emotional danger, explains much, but it cannot be regarded as being a complete answer to the question: 'What is the meaning of pain?' Many people have tried to find in suffering some deeper and spiritual significance. The more primitive religions definitely taught that pain was a punishment inflicted by an outraged deity, and the less primitive considered it to be a means of discipline. Hinton, well known as the author of a book published at the end of the last century and entitled, *The Mystery of Pain*, wrote on this subject. A strongly religious man, as well as a distinguished surgeon, he believed that pain had some spiritual significance and that it must be regarded as an aid to man's spiritual development. He points out that payment is a principle in life, and that many of our pleasures are enhanced by the fact that we have paid for them by suffering. A strong and healthy man engaged in a hard day's hunting absorbs into his pleasure a large amount of what a weak person would consider to be unbearable fatigue and discomfort. The experiences which a weak man would regard as intolerable for the sportsman become the very conditions which determine his enjoyment. Hinton looks upon childbirth as providing a still more striking example of pain enhancing an emotion; the mother accepts without questioning the pains of labour and by this acceptance it is generally believed that her love for her child is deepened. This view seems to be supported by the experiments made by E. N. Marais and reported in his work, *The Soul of the White Ant*. Using the Kaffir buck of South Africa for his experiments he anaesthetized six of these animals during labour. In all six cases the mother subsequently refused to accept her lamb for suckling. To prove that the refusal was not due to the general disturbance caused by the anaesthetic Marais chloroformed six Kaffir does immediately after delivery, but before they had seen their lambs. These six mothers behaved like normal mothers and readily accepted their offspring. From these and from other experiments Marais concludes that without pain there can be no mother love in nature. To what extent these results of animal experiments are applicable to human beings must be a matter of doubt, but they undoubtedly lend some support to the view that a mother's love is deepened by the suffering of childbirth.

Keats shared Hinton's view that pain and suffering may be instrumental in helping man's spiritual development. In a letter to his brother, the poet wrote:

> I will call the *world* a School instituted for the purpose of teaching little children to read — I will call the human heart the horn Book read in the School — and I will call the *child able to read* the Soul made from the *School* and its *horn book*. Do you not see how

necessary a *World* of Pains and troubles is to school an Intelligence and make it a Soul. A place where the heart must feel and suffer in a thousand diverse ways . . . As various as the Lives of Men are — so various become their Souls, and thus does God make individual beings, Souls, Identical Souls of the sparks of his own essence. This appears to me a faint sketch of a system of Salvation which does not offend our reason and humanity.

Gerald Heard, like Hinton and Keats, links up pain with an evolutionary process in man, but in an entirely different and, to my way of thinking, unsatisfactory manner. Man, says Heard, is in process of spiritual evolution, for which a store of energy is required. 'Pain', he asserts, 'is a measure, if a crude one, of the degree of vital creative energy in any creature, animal or man' Unless the creative energy within us be expended in the work for which it was intended, namely, evolution, it is liable to manifest itself as pain. According to this author:

The more mentally active anyone is, the less he is capable of pain.

An attack of pain, therefore, in Heard's opinion, should be regarded as a warning of the misuse of our latent creative energy:

Pain is a violent intermittent warning that we should spend and not hoard the most valuable gift any being could possess, the energy required for growth in awareness, for creative evolutionary development.

In advancing this view Heard makes two unwarrantable assumptions: the first that an evolutionary process is actually taking place in man, and the second that pain is a manifestation of the misuse of energy required for it. No justification can be found for either of these two assumptions. Whatever may be said of certain individuals, there exists not the slightest evidence of any automatic spiritual progress amongst men in general. Mark Twain wrote:

From everlasting to everlasting, this is the law: the *sum* of wrong and misery shall always keep step with the sum of human blessedness. No civilization, no advance, has ever modified these propositions by even the shadow of a shade, nor ever can while our race endures. (*What is Man?*)

If this be so, and I believe that Mark Twain wrote truly, Heard's subsidiary theory that pain is an indication of misapplied creative energy is entirely without basis. It should be noted that although Hinton, like Heard, associates pain with the idea of spiritual evolution, he does not assume the existence of any automatic progress of man. All that he claims is that pain may be usefully employed by certain individuals in their struggle to achieve spiritual development. Whilst Heard implies that if we feel no pain we are probably evolving, Hinton tells us that if we use our pain properly we may gain a spiritual reward.

Keats considers a world of pain and trouble as necessary to our salvation, and there can be little doubt that nothing less compelling than pain has the power to rouse us from our trance. Life hypnotizes us, our possessions and our activities enthral us, and we are old without having given more than a passing thought to the why and the wherefore of our existence. But sometimes pain and suffering can interrupt for a short spell this headlong career through life and compel us to wonder what it all means. By their action we may be forced for a moment to stop and face the issues from which all our life we have been escaping. A sharp attack of cardiac pain accompanied by a struggle for breath, and our world sways, breaks and falls apart, revealing the stern realities which we would not see. As the pain recedes we find ourselves staring at the same old familiar things, the pattern on the counterpane, the shaded light in the bedroom, the picture on the wall opposite, but somehow, all of them have lost their solidity They have become thin and as unsubstantial as stage properties seen by daylight. During those long-drawn-out agonizing minutes through which we have just passed, the spheres of life and death have merged and even although, in the end, it was death which withdrew, in that withdrawal it has taken with it a few of our poor illusions. Life may never be quite the same for us afterwards. Soon the play will be resumed and the actor in us will continue to strut and speak, but with perhaps a little less confidence than before. If the realization has been deep enough, we may remember that we are moving amidst painted boards and canvas, and that once against a background of fear and pain we viewed the stark realities of life and death. After such an experience the world may indeed become a School, and the heart its hornbook. It may be that R. L. Stevenson had in mind the hypnotic action which life exercises over us, and the gradual weakening in us of the capacity to feel real emotions when he wrote the poem, *Celestial Surgeon*:

> O Lord, if too obdurate I
> Choose Thou before that spirit die,
> A piercing pain, a killing sin,
> And to my dead heart run them in!

Life is so insistent and the spirit is so swathed about with its petty cares and pleasures that at an early age it may cease to grow. As the intuitive genius of Keats clearly understood, a measure of pain and suffering may be necessary for its salvation. They are capable of teaching us patience and forbearance, and this was the lesson Job learnt. 'What shall I answer Thee?' he cried to the God who had tested him with tribulation. 'I will lay my hand upon my mouth.' But all do not learn the same lesson. Some only learn anger and selfishness, bitterness and despair.

CHAPTER V

THE PROBLEMS OF OLD AGE

IN Bede's parable life is likened to the flight of a bird across a lighted room, in through the window of birth and out again through the window of death into the darkness from which it came. For a few fleeting moments it is here, and then it is gone. A hundred different sayings remind us of life's brevity; innumerable poems have for their theme the transiency of all our possessions. Beauty fades, strength departs and with gathering speed old age approaches. We see it in the faces of our friends before we note it in our own; half of the world grows older, half grows younger whilst we remain the same. I am continually surprised by the increasing youth of the police force and by the boyish faces I meet in the courtyard when I visit my old college at Cambridge. For a time we succeed in deluding ourselves that we are younger than our years, but in the end we are forced to accept the evidence supplied by our mirrors and by the candour of our friends; we also have graduated from youth and are amongst the middle aged. Most of us accept the discovery ungraciously, and with a sense of grievance. It is not so much that we protest against the fate that finally awaits us as that we recoil from the deterioration of faculties which precedes it. If we were birds making a graceful swoop across a room, we would accept our sudden disappearance philosophically, but we are birds moulting feathers and staggering in our flight. It is the ignominious departure, the gracelessness of our exit, which disturb us.

In no place is this silent protest against old age more apparent than in the consulting-room. Because each decade of life has its appropriate illnesses, it is customary, when taking a patient's history, to inquire his age. It is always interesting to note a patient's reaction to the question: 'How old are you?' For the young it brings no embarrassment; the reply comes promptly. The middle aged usually answer after a momentary hesitation, and often add the rider that they certainly do not feel as old as this, indeed, no older than they were ten years ago. The old either look gloomy, or else smile, and the smile may be followed by the response, 'Guess what my age is?' The words come gleefully and with an overtone of challenge. Being something of a diplomatist the medical man ventures a glaring understatement, and the little comedy closes in an atmosphere of mingled surprise and delight. The protest against advancing years is partly due to our limited conception of life and time. We see our life, that is to say, our time, as a line along which we are being relentlessly pushed in a direction in which we have no desire to go. Unwilling travellers, we look back with longing to a past glorified and freed of all associated disadvantages by our imagination. Contrasted with the highly coloured 'then', the 'now' appears.drab, and, like children who have been given a shabby and unwanted toy, we look at it askance. Even though the 'now' also has inherent merits, they are not to our liking. What are maturity and experience compared with that which we appear to have lost?

This way of thinking on the subject of age is peculiar to Europe and America, and is not necessarily typical of mankind as a whole. In contrasting Eastern and Western cultures, Lin Yutang says that he found very little difference between Western nations and his own country, China, in their attitude to sex, women, work, play, liberty and democracy, but a marked difference in their attitude to age.

> In China, the first question a person asks the other on an official call, after asking about his name and surname, is, 'What is your glorious age?' If the person replies apologetically that he is twenty-three or twenty-eight, the other party generally comforts him that he has still a glorious future, and that one day he may become old. But if the person replies that he is thirty-five or thirty-eight, the other party immediately exclaims with deep respect, 'Good luck!'; enthusiasm grows in proportion as a gentleman is able to report a higher and higher age, and if the person is anywhere over fifty, the inquirer immediately drops his voice in humility and respect. That is why all old people, if they can, should go and live in China, where even a beggar with a white beard is treated with extra kindness. (LIN YUTANG: *The Importance of Living*.)

This difference between the East and the West is readily understandable. Chinese society has its roots in family life, and in the Chinese home the old mother and father are honoured figures. The West is enamoured of individual independence, and family life is slowly disappearing. But there is a still more important reason for the European's and the American's distaste for old age. Because in the West such high value is placed on activity, a diminished capacity for action makes a man feel that he is on the downward slope of life's journey. If he were truly consistent in this view, he should begin to deplore this decline in the mid-twenties, for tests carried out in America have shown that the zenith of muscular activity and endurance coincide with the age of twenty-two or twenty-three. From this age onwards the physical efficiency of the body slowly declines, dropping more swiftly after the fortieth year has been reached. But man's mind and spirit grow more slowly than does his body, and since the East reverences wisdom and experience rather than activity, age is accepted gladly. In China the old man with 'ruddy cheeks and white hair' is looked upon as being the symbol of ultimate earthly happiness.

In calculating our length of life we use the unit of measurement which man has found to be the most convenient, namely, the year, or the time taken for the earth to make a complete circuit of the sun; we state, for example, that the life of a certain man corresponds in duration to eighty revolutions of the earth round the sun. In making this comparison we are measuring one kind of motion by reference to another, and the measuring-rod we have selected for this purpose has the advantage of remaining constant. But, as Carrel has emphasized in *Man, the Unknown*, there exists for all living creatures an internal, as well as an external, measurement of living, which he calls 'inner time'. This inner time is not measured by any external standard but by the changes which take place in the body during the course of a life. Like external, or solar time, this inner time may be thought of as a movement, or as a succession of organic and of mental states. Some of the changes which mark this movement are rhythmic and reversible, for example, the beat of the heart, inspiration and expiration, the contraction and relaxation of muscles, the alternate states of activity and rest in the various glands of the body and in digestion, and the ebb and flow of menstruation. Other changes which measure inner time are non-rhythmic and irreversible, such as the gradual loss of the skin's elasticity, the diminution in the transparency of the lens, the atrophy of glandular structures, and the slow hardening of the tissues with increasing age. But whether rhythmic or non-rhythmic, reversible or irreversible, the speed of these changes varies in different people and at different ages; sometimes the inner movements are accelerated and sometimes they are retarded. Because of these fluctuations in speed, inner time does not necessarily synchronize with external time, that is to say, with the solar measuring-rod which we have selected for determining the length of our life. Sometimes the inner clock moves faster and sometimes it moves slower, and the discrepancy between inner and outer time is often very great, so great that it cannot be lightly dismissed as a matter of purely academic interest. For example, in the hibernating animal the organic changes which give the measurement of inner time are so slowed down that they seem almost to have stopped, and in a dried rotifer inner time may be said to have actually stopped. Only with the approach of spring does the inner clock of the rotifer begin to move again, gathering speed as the days grow warmer and accelerating to a maximum with the arrival of summer.

These changes in the speed of the inner time of an organism are physiological, and vary with the conditions under which the organism lives. But scientists have shown that it is possible also to accelerate or retard the inner clock artificially. By keeping flies at an abnormally high temperature, Loeb speeded up this inner time so effectively that he brought about in them premature ageing.[1] His treated flies undoubtedly lived more intensely than their fellows, but judged by external standards they died before 'their time'. Human beings are more conscious than flies and because of this we are able to judge the rate of our inner time, not only by the speed of bodly changes, but also by means of psychological phenomena. Consciousness makes us aware of psychic processes and we can note the speed with which one impression is replaced by another, in other words the speed of psychological time. When we say that time flies, or that it drags, we are referring to the psychological clock by which duration may be measured. We can all recall occasions when we received so many

---

[1] Francois carried out somewhat similar experiments in human beings. After having instructed his subjects to strike a Morse key at what they estimated to be the rate of three times a second, he raised their body temperatures by means of a diathermy current. The rise in body temperature speeded up all physical and psychic processes, and the subjects of his experiment struck the Morse key far more rapidly. Physiological and psychological time had been changed for them (*Biological Time*).

impressions that looking at our watches afterwards we were surprised that only an hour of solar time had passed. We can also remember other occasions when impressions were so dulled that we appeared to have lived only for a few moments, and yet our watches have recorded the passage of an hour. The speed of psychological time changes in different states of consciousness and at different periods of our lives. Within the course of a summer's day a child may record so many vivid impressions and experience such a wealth of emotions that no day of adult life would be long enough to contain them. The child stretches out time so that the minutes become hours, the hours days, the days weeks. In old age the reverse happens; the old man feels and senses so little that his inner clock seems to be running down, and external time to be quickening its pace. He sits by the fireside for hours with old memories stirring within him, only dimly conscious of what is happening around him and dreaming away the store of time which still remains to him. When working on the rate of the cicatrization of wounds at the Rockefeller Institute Carrel found that the amount of solar time required by a man of fifty to effect a certain unit of repair was about five times more than that required by a child of ten. For the man of fifty solar time flowed four times faster.

And as Loeb and others have been able to alter the rhythm of inner changes in their laboratory animals, so can we by artificial means, such as the taking of drugs, change the tempo of our impressions. A speeding up of psychic processes is experienced in states of heightened consciousness, in the moments of illumination described by saints and seers and occasionally under the influence of anaesthetics.

We are in possession therefore of two standards by which to measure life: an external measuring-rod provided by the sun, and an internal standard which, because it is our own, is actually more important to us. Long life is not a matter of surviving many years, but of living as richly and fully as lies within our power. The biologist Child, by alternately feeding and starving flat-worms, was able to arrest their growth, so that they remained stationary, whilst control worms, not so treated, were passing through nineteen generations. Measured by external time the lives of Child's worms were prolonged far beyond their natural span, but measured by their own inner time they lived no longer than did their fellows. Loeb carried out similar experiments on sea urchins' eggs; by lowering the temperature to 10° C. he extended the life of the eggs a thousandfold. Apples can also be preserved almost indefinitely by carefully lowering their temperature, and later, when they are required for eating, raising it with equal care. Such apples are not so much preserved as maintained in a state of suspended life. It is interesting to speculate what might happen if this process were so perfected that it could be applied with safety to animals and even to human beings. We can imagine a man deciding to withdraw from the troubles of the present years by retiring for a time into cold storage, leaving instructions that he should be unfrozen when the war was ended and the world had settled down. If his instructions were successfully carried out, and he returned to active existence after, say, fifteen years of suspended animation, such a man would have increased the duration of his life as measured by external solar time, but by his own inner time he would have lived no longer. Life cannot be measured in terms of years but only in terms of inner experience.

The changes in the tissues which accompany age have been submitted during the last twenty years to an intensive study, and the question has often been debated whether they are pathological or physiological. In other words: Is old age a disease, or is it the inevitable lot of all living creatures? Even this simple question has not been finally answered. Leo Loeb, an expert in tissue culture experiments, has summed up his opinion in the following words:

> All the essential tissues of the metazoan body are potentially immortal . . . It is the differentiation of function of mutually dependent aggregates of cells and tissues which constitute the metazoan body, which brings about death, and no inherent or inevitable mortal process in the individual cells themselves.

Death, therefore, according to Loeb, is the price we pay for our complexity, and many of the inner disturbances, producing illness, are due to the same cause. Cultures from the heart of an embryo chick started by Carrel in 1912 are still being kept alive in the Rockefeller Institute. But it must be borne in mind that the cells of this tissue have survived by means of ceaseless division. Their longevity therefore is that of the race, and not that of an individual, for as individuals the original cells which made up this tissue have long ceased to exist. It is true that by giving up all to their children they have left behind no corpse, and have thus escaped the processes of decay, but they are immortal only through their descendants. They are in the same category as the germinal cells in our bodies which by becoming our children avoid destruction.

Even when we confine our attention to simple unicellular organisms, their youth, as measured by their power to divide, would appear to be subject to certain limitations. Catkin and Child, experimenting with protozoa, state that although cell division can continue a long time, in the end it slows down and appears to become more and more difficult. When this happens an interesting phenomenon is observed: two of the protozoa come together and fuse into a single individual. This act of conjugation has a rejuvenating action, and increases the capacity of the fused couple to divide. It is not necessary for either of them to be young in order that this may happen, a rejuvenating action is noted even when both cells are equally elderly. It is the interchange in material between them which is responsible for the increase in their vigour. These observations suggest two things: first, that even unicellular organisms are subject to old age, and second, that when this overtakes them they have the power to restore their youth by a process of rejuvenation.

Can the lesson which has been learnt from the study of protozoa be applied to man? Can a man be rejuvenated? It is obvious that an invigorating action brought about by conjugation is inapplicable to human beings. The complexity of the structure of the higher animals, let alone of man, excludes the possibility of such a simple method of rejuvenation. In Langdon Brown's picturesque phrase, 'to play general post now would be to reduce the whole body to chaos'. Before discussing what alternative method of rejuvenation might be applicable to multicellular organisms and to man, it is first necessary to understand clearly what we mean by the word 'rejuvenation'. What is usually meant by this term is really a reversal of inner time; the changes which time has wrought in the body of the ageing man are reversed, and he is carried back to a previous stage of his life. Somewhat inconsistently we generally suppose that the rejuvenated secretions and tissues would still retain their memories; the brain would become young without sacrificing its wisdom and experience. It is obvious that a complete reversal of inner processes of this kind is a very different matter from the slowing down of the inner clocks of flat-worms and sea urchins' eggs effected by Child and Loeb. A true rejuvenation would entail a marked change in the structure and chemical composition of the body cells. Bechhold has shown that the diminishing power of cells to reproduce themselves which we have taken as a criterion of age is associated with the loss of their affinity for water. The older the cell the less water does it contain; whereas the water content of the cells of the foetus is 94 per cent, and of the new-born child 70 per cent, that of the ageing man is only 50 per cent. It would be possible, therefore, to express the difference between the Archbishop of Canterbury and his youngest chorister in terms of water, as well as in terms of years, the Primate containing only 50 per cent of water and the chorister about 65 per cent. This progressive dehydration is responsible for the elderly man's loss of elasticity, and for the hardening of his tissues, and if a true rejuvenation is to be effected a change in the colloid of the cell would have to be effected. What is of particular interest is that the hardening and loss of elasticity of the body of an old man are associated with what may be regarded as being corresponding changes in his psychic functions. The mind of an aged man has lost all its resilience. It is like a tablet of wax which has become brittle and hard and is no longer able to receive impressions. What is already marked upon it is retained, but it is useless for the inscription of any new messages. New scenes and new experiences may still be registered, but because they are immediately related to the deeper impressions of the past, the memory of them is seldom retained. It is not surprising that old people are lacking in resilience, and find it difficult to adjust themselves to new conditions. Their bodies have lost their elasticity and their minds are graven only with the images of the past.

The search for the Elixir of Life is of such antiquity, and so many attempts have been made to find it, that it will be necessary to deal with the subject of rejuvenation in greater detail.

CHAPTER VI

REJUVENATION

To survey the medical literature of rejuvenation is to follow the progress of medicine and of science throughout the ages. Every change in the fundamental doctrine of medicine has diverted the general direction of the search for the Elixir of Life. When the doctrine of the four cardinal humours of the body was an article of medical faith, it was believed that the body would be invigorated if the sanguine humour could be reinforced. 'Blood', wrote Goethe in *Faust:* 'is a very special fluid', and all through the ages magical properties have been accredited to it. It is recorded that an attempt was made to rejuvenate Innocent VIII along these lines by transfusing him with the blood of three youths. The Holy Father's death shortly after the completion of this difficult operation cannot be taken as a proof that this belief was wrong. It is explained by the fact that the technique of transfusion was at that time extremely imperfect, and that nothing was known about the incompatibility of different types of blood. With a better technique the aged Pope might well have benefited from the treatment he received. Modern science even lends support to the view that the choice of young donors was a wise one. Recently it has been shown that tissue cultures grow better in blood which has been taken from youthful animals. This suggests that young blood contains some substance which has a stimulating action on cell division. Ischloudsky's work indicates that this substance exists not only in the blood, but also in all youthful tissues. For many years this scientist has been attempting to rejuvenate old animals by means of extracts obtained from the tissues of embryo calves. The full results of his treatment have not yet been published, but the preliminary reports issued by Ischlondsky contain a great deal of interesting reading. It must be remembered, however, that the success of any form of rejuvenation treatment depends, to a great extent, on whether the changes that have occurred in the ageing body are still capable of being reversed. If they have progressed beyond a certain stage and the vitality of the cells has been irreparably damaged, no form of treatment can be expected to prove effective. There is a point beyond which all changes, biological or chemical, become irreversible.

When, towards the close of the last century, the ductless glands began to yield up their secrets, the attention of the medical profession was immediately turned in this direction. The discovery of the active principle of the thyroid, and the miracles wrought by it in cases of thyroid deficiency, soon encouraged the idea that further progress in endocrinology would result in the discovery of the long-sought-for Elixir of Life. Because of a certain superficial resemblance between the old man and the eunuch, particular hopes were entertained of the sex glands and there were not a few who believed that eventually from these glands would be obtained some extract capable of restoring vitality to the ageing body. So long ago as 1869 Brown-Séquard had announced that his own health had been so benefited by injecting himself with crude extracts of the testes of dogs, that he had been enabled to continue his work long after he had been on the point of retiring on account of his age. None of his contemporaries had accepted these experiments as a proof of the existence of an invigorating principle in the testes, but now that organotherapy had become fashionable, his words were remembered. Steinach, a Viennese physiologist, determined to follow the lead which Brown-Séquard had given, and made a great number of experiments on aged animals. Because no chemist had succeeded at that time in extracting an active principle from the testes, he instituted a new method of treatment, namely, ligature of the *vas deferens*, or duct leading from the testicle. Steinach postulated that by putting out of action the external function of the gland, that is to say, the formation of semen, its activity would be entirely concentrated on the internal function, namely, the production of an internal secretion. A few years later he claimed that by means of this simple operation he had succeeded in rejuvenating a number of aged laboratory animals. He now advocated its application to man.

Twenty years have elapsed since Steinach published his researches, and the operation of vaso-ligature has been performed on thousands of human beings. We are now in a position to assess the value of this form of treatment. It must be confessed that although quite a number of patients have believed themselves to have benefited from the Steinach operation, no satisfactory objective evidence of rejuvenation has been obtained. The fact that a man has submitted to a wonderful operation has a strong effect on his imagination, and this alone would be sufficient to account for much of the improvement which has been noted. Not only is there no satisfactory evidence by means of which a patient's statements can be corroborated, but the scientific basis of Steinach's work is now considered doubtful. It is by no means certain that the output of internal secretion is increased by ligaturing the duct. In any case, the recent isolation of the active principle of the testis has obviated the necessity of resorting to the operation of vaso-ligature. Injections of a potent extract can now be given, and the results of flooding the blood-stream with 'male hormone' directly observed.

At the time when Steinach was employing vaso-ligature in Vienna, Voronoff, working on the same theory, namely, that senility is due to failure of the internal secretion of the sex glands, was making use of testicular grafts. From the very beginning scientists were sceptical of Voronoff's work, for they knew that when tissues from the lower animals are grafted on to a man, they are rapidly absorbed; the human body resents the presence of cells taken from another species, and, regarding them as foreign material, promptly destroys them. Voronoff believed that he could avoid this difficulty by making use of grafts taken from man's nearest relatives, the higher apes, and proceeded with his work. Soon he began to make extravagant claims to brilliant results obtained from his testicular implants, claims which the scientific world as a whole did not accept. I have myself performed Voronoff's operation many times, employing grafts from human testicles which had to be removed because they were misplaced and were causing inconvenience. Since few of these human grafts survived for longer than a year, I cannot accept Voronoff's statement that tissue taken from a chimpanzee fares any better. Even Voronoff's work on aged animals, in which grafting material from the same species was used, must be regarded as having given doubtful results. A report drawn up in 1928 by a special committee of experts appointed by the French Government to investigate Voronoff's claims produced the following guarded verdict:

The claims of Dr. Voronoff to effect rejuvenation of the aged and decrepit male by testicular grafting is possibly justifiable. The evidence is, however, not based on critical experimentation.

In spite of the doubts expressed by scientists, Steinach's and Voronoff's work gained great publicity and hundreds of elderly patients flocked to the consulting-rooms of the rejuvenation specialists in the hope of regaining their youth. Those who were able to pay large fees visited Paris and were treated by Voronoff himself. Rumour has it that on the eve of his marriage an elderly British millionaire summoned the Paris expert to London. The great man, accompanied by a chimpanzee, arrived at one of London's smartest hotels, where he was greeted by the bride and bridegroom, and later by two distinguished English physicians. After a preliminary conference the operation was performed. As is, perhaps, only natural, the result of it was not made public.

Steinach and Voronoff's methods of rejuvenation do not rest on any secure scientific foundation. Old age, as we have seen, is associated with profound changes in all the body tissues, changes which it is impossible to attribute to the failure of a single gland. Even if the activity of *all* the endocrine glands could be revived, it is doubtful whether this would have the effect of reversing the dehydration of colloids associated with old age, and if any *one* of the glands is to be selected for treatment it should undoubtedly be the pituitary rather than the sex glands. The pituitary is the master of the ductless glands, and an increased action on its part would be more likely to have a widespread action on the body.

A more promising line of attack on old age is offered by the prompt treatment of the pathological conditions which accompany it. Even such characteristic changes as loss of elasticity, atrophy of organs, and the replacement of higher tissues by connective tissue, are not necessarily brought about by age, but may be the result of disease. Rossli reports the existence of advanced old-age changes in a youth of seventeen and in a girl of fifteen. Some pathological factor must have existed which was responsible for the premature senility of these two adolescents. Ischlondsky asserts that death is more often due to pathological than to physiological factors; in other words he believes that the majority of people die before their time. In his opinion the duration of human life is longer than the three score and ten years allotted by the psalmist, and in support of this view he cites the disproportion between the longevity of the psychic and of the vegetative functions of man. As a rule people die before their psychic faculties have deteriorated.

> It is sufficient [Ischlondsky states] to recall the innumerable cases of death of great intellectuals, scientists, philosophers, to notice the striking difference between the psychical condition of these people at the moment of death, and the physical failure which caused death.

And even when the psychic functions have deteriorated, this deterioration is generally due to a failure of the circulation through the brain, in other words, to a failure of a secondary vegetative function. When Ischlondsky enumerates what he believes to be the causes of this premature death, he gives an important place to the emotional factors which have been discussed at length in Chapter III. Excessive and prolonged emotional activity produces a marked inhibition of functions which are of the greatest importance, or which are even indispensable to the harmonious life of the organism as a whole.

> But if the excitation of the cortical centres becomes more or less continual — which is undoubtedly the case in regard to most of the higher nervous centres owing to the very complicated conditions of contemporary psychical life — the inhibition of other centres becomes practically constant, determining a lowering of many important vegetative functions, a diminution of assimilation and dissimilation, a decrease of the metabolism of the various physiological systems and, at last, a precocious senility with all its characteristic signs. .(N. E. ISCHLONDSKY: *Protoformotherapy*.)

If Ischlondsky be right, attempts to combat the changes brought about by old age cannot be looked upon as being a struggle against the laws of nature, but rather as a struggle against the laws of man. Because we live wrongly, we die prematurely.

A century ago, when Oliver Wendell Holmes was asked the way to attain long life, he replied: 'Some years before birth advertise for a couple of parents both belonging to long-lived families.' His recipe for long life could not be bettered. When centenarians are interviewed and asked for the secret of their longevity, they give a great variety of answers, many of which are inconsistent; some have always been temperate and some have always lived well, some like their 'beer and baccy', some are hearty eaters, and others eat but sparingly; no help can be obtained from their answers. If, however, their family histories be investigated, it will almost always be found that they come of long-lived stock. Professor Raymond Pearl and his associates at Johns Hopkins University have collected the pedigrees of 365 nonagenarians, and have found that the average life-span of their parents was from twelve to seventeen years longer than that of the parents of an un-selected group of people. One centenarian was found to be descended from parents who had lived to be 97 and 101, and from grandparents of 104, 98, 106 and 93. Pearl believes that long-lived people survive because they have inherited 'organically superior constitutions resistant to infection'. They have also been born with the capacity to adjust to unfavourable environmental factors, such as infections, work and poisons. Emotional stability was a predominant trait amongst nonagenarians and centenarians; the great majority of them were of 'a placid temperament, not given to worry. They had taken life at an even, unhurried pace. The length of life is generally in inverse propor-tion to the rate of living — the more rapid the pace, the shorter the time that life endures'.

Among the methods which have been advocated for the combating of the pathological changes associated with age must be mentioned the sour milk' treatment of Metchnikoff. This Russian scientist noticed that the proportion of centenarians was high amongst Bulgarian drinkers of 'koumis'. He was of the opinion that the lactic acid bacillus which brings about the souring of milk altered the reaction of the bowel, and thereby eliminated some of the noxious bacteria which it harboured. He postulated that the poisons produced by these bacteria were responsible for some of the degenerative changes that occurred in the body. But Metchnikoff's treatment of old age embraced more than the taking of sour milk. He expounded the philosophy of 'orthobiosis', in plain terms, of correct living, believing that it was not only man's body, but his spirit which determined the length of his life.

Metchnikoff was right to emphasize the importance of right living in the attainment of long life. Motorists know that if they drive un-skilfully, jerking their gears, accelerating, 'driving on their brakes' and straining the engines on hills, their cars will soon wear out. Yet the same motorists who avoid all unnecessary wear and tear on their cars seldom stop to consider how they are manipulating the machinery of their own minds and bodies. Few of us seek for a technique of living or deem it necessary to seek for one. We assume that we know all about ourselves, and that, in any case, nature has endowed us with instincts which teach us all that it is necessary to know. To learn a technique of right living seems, therefore, to be superfluous. And yet, if the truth were known, we understand ourselves far less than we understand our cars, and are more in need of instruction in living than in driving. Practical instruction in living was formerly a branch of religious teaching, as exemplified by the Tao of ancient China. For five centuries before the coming of Christ the followers of Lao Tze studied and sought to live in conformity with the laws of nature, adopting what has sometimes been called the principle of non-angularity. Tranquil in mind and healthy in body, the Taoists attained such ripe ages that it was generally supposed that they had discovered the Elixir of Life. The Emperor Chi-Hoang-Ti (221-209 B.C.) was so impressed by their longevity that he determined to discover their secret. Having been told of some islands known only to the Taoists, where a beverage was brewed which conferred immortality on man, he equipped a special expedition to search for them. But the secret of the Taoists' long life did not lie in any magic formula. They held that the man whose manner of life and behaviour was in conformity with Tao, the Way of Nature, would attain the attributes of Tao This belief was crystallized in the saying:

> Possessed of Tao, he endures long; to the end of his bodily life he is exempt from danger and decay.

The dictum that a man's manner of life and behaviour must be in conformity with nature has many meanings, amongst others that each phase of life has its own significance and its appropriate activities. Childhood must be looked upon as being a period of active growth, not only of the body, but also of the mind. By means of play the child prepares himself for the sterner realities of life with which he will have to deal later on. At puberty the pace of development is quickened, and in youth a true apprenticeship to life begins. Maturity brings with it increasing responsibilities, and it is during this stage of life that a man is called upon to establish himself in the world, marry and rear a family. With the beginning of old age these responsibilities are lightened. Havelock Ellis writes of this period of a man's life as follows:

> With the coming of age the burden falls away. All the anxieties and responsibilities have become light; even if work remains practice has made it easy. He is no longer a timid stranger in an unfamiliar world, full of obscure terrors, no longer tortured to find his own path . . . It becomes possible to understand the saying of Plutarch, that the mind becomes youthful in advancing years. (HAVELOCK ELLIS: *Questions of our Time.*)

In primitive civilizations the older members of the community form the tribal council and are the repository of its traditions and its wisdom, and in less primitive civilizations they become the elder statesmen, the advisers and counsellors. In the East, which has always placed more emphasis on the cultivation of wisdom than on worldly activity, men who have reached this stage often leave their homes to lead a life of contemplation and religious devotion. Each phase of life has its appropriate activities and meaning, and we can be certain that a human being would not survive to the age of seventy or eighty unless his survival served some purpose. Nature is too economical to allow a man to encumber the ground if a decline in his physical powers renders him superfluous and useless.

Much has been made of the difficulties of the passage from childhood to adult life, but far less emphasis has been placed on the equally difficult passage from maturity to old age. Many psychologists have described the disposition shown by certain children to shrink back at the threshold of adult life and to take refuge in infantile fantasies. Few psychologists have spoken of the many men and women who recoil from entering what they allow themselves to think of as being the grey and chill country of old age. Jung is one of the few modern psychologists who has written on this subject with sympathy and understanding. He feels that the difficulties caused by advancing years weigh so heavily on many people that special schools for adults would seem to be necessary, schools in which they may be prepared for the new responsibilities which await them:

I said just now that we have no schools for forty-year-olds.
That is not quite true. Our religions were always such schools in
the past, but how many people regard them as such to-day? How
many of us older persons have really been brought up in such a
school, and prepared for the second half of life, for old age, death
and eternity? (C. C. JUNG: *Modern Man in Search of a Soul.*)

Because life seems meaningless and because during their more active
years they have been entirely engrossed in their businesses, their pro-
fessions and their amusements, retirement is for many men a time of
anxiety and danger. Their inability to continue doing what they have
always done leads such men to believe that their day is over. By means
of newspapers, bridge and golf they continue to eke out a few tedious
years and then, having no motive for living, they quietly die.

> The best antidote against senile decay [wrote Sir James Crichton-
> Browne, himself a striking example of a green old age] is an active
> interest in human affairs, and those keep young longest who love
> most.

Michelangelo, Titian, Cellini, Metchnikoff, Tolstoi, Pavlov and Chief
Justice Wendell Holmes bear witness to the truth of this saying. In
writing of the importance of activity, both mental and physical, in
keeping the body young, Sir Humphrey Rolleston quotes Lytton
Strachey's description of the circle in which Mme du Deffand moved:

> They refused to grow old; they almost refused to die. Time,
> himself, seems to have joined their circle, to have been infected
> with their politeness, and to have absolved them, to the furthest
> possible point, from the operation of his laws: Voltaire, D'Argen-
> tal, Moncrif, Henault, Madame d'Egmont, Mme du Deffand
> herself, all lived to be well over eighty, with the full zest of their
> activities unimpaired.

Longevity is not a question of miraculous draughts, or diets, or
hormones, or grafts, but of right living, both of the body and of the
mind. If we would live longer, we must first learn to live better.
Compared to the animals, the natural span of our life is a generous one,
but too often we squander our inheritance and die before our time.

CHAPTER VII

DEATH AND DYING

METCHNIKOFF tells us that when Tolstoi wanted to write about death and turned to the scientific literature of his time in order to find out what scientists had to say about it, he was distressed by how little he could find. Scientists appeared to take but little interest in a subject which had always been of supreme importance to religious men, philosophers and poets. Death for the scientists was, as Faber has since said, 'an unsurveyed land'. Tolstoi lived at the height of the industrial age, the era of mechanistic thought, and if, having failed to find what he wanted in literature, he had asked a contemporary biologist for an explanation of death, he would have been told that death was the result of the wearing out of the body; it represented the final break in an old piece of machinery. This false picture of death has now been abandoned, for life can no longer be thought of in terms of machinery. Unlike an engine, the body has the capacity to renew itself continuously by the building up of new material into its tissues. This being so, it need not wear out until the limit of the cells' capacity to reproduce themselves has been reached. Life is dependent on growth, and only that which continues to reproduce itself can survive. What grows most vigorously avoids death most successfully. In a dynamic universe nothing can remain stationary; it must either advance or retreat, grow or decay. Although the capacity of cells to reproduce themselves may not be unlimited, they can go on dividing for a very long time. This is more especially the case amongst organisms, such as trees, in which no narrow limit has been placed on the size which they may attain.

Trees are the longest lived of all the creatures which inhabit the earth; they are the veterans of organic life. Metchnikoff describes a gigantic dragon-tree in Teneriffe which was so old that it had become a local tutelary deity. Even when the island was first discovered in the fifteenth century this venerable giant had long been an object of worship. Humboldt, who wrote about it in 1808, stated that its trunk measured 45 ft. in circumference. Since dragon-trees are slow growing, this means that even at that time it must have been of immense antiquity. In 1819 a tempest swept over the island and a third of its foliage came crashing to the ground. In spite of this disaster and of further damage done by subsequent storms, it was not until 1868 that Teneriffe's ancient deity was finally overthrown. Similar examples of long life in trees are provided by this country, many of our old yews having been planted in the twelfth century in order to supply wood for the famous English long-bow. But it is to the New World that we must go for the greatest veterans amongst trees. In the red-wood forests of California are trees believed to be thousands of years old.

But the linking up of death with failure in growth adds but little to our knowledge of it. Just as it was necessary to turn from the individual life, to life as a whole, in order to understand the nature of disease, so must we study the larger unit in order to find the significance of death. J. B. S. Haldane writes of death as follows:

> So far as we can at present understand the matter, the physiology of death, and that of reproductive and social activity in all their wide ramifications, belong to the physiology of the species. The individual organism, like the individual cell in a complex organism, belongs to a wider organic whole, apart from which much of its life is unintelligible.

I do not agree that the physiology of the species throws any light on death's meaning. Biologists have been repeating Darwin's famous phrase, 'the survival of the fittest', ever since this great master first uttered it, and it was inevitable that they should look upon death as nature's method of eliminating the unfit and of thus improving the general stock. But death does its work so blindly that it cannot be regarded as a satisfactory agent by the eugenists. Too often the unhealthy survive whilst the active and healthy, because they take risks which an invalid would avoid, perish. It is only by relating death to a larger unit than that to which Haldane refers us, namely, to organic life as a whole, that any meaning can be found for it.

We have seen that organic life may be looked upon as being an integrated organism to which individual organisms are related much as individual cells are related to the body. And as it is impossible to consider the life-history of a cell without reference to the greater being of which it forms a part, so is it impossible to consider the life and death of an organism without reference to the aggregate of organic life. Life is nourished by life and in turn supports life, and when the time of the individual comes to an end, whether it be that of the cell or of the organism, the organism returns to that greater being from which it came. By means of ciné-photography and tissue culture we can witness on the screen the life-history of body cells. We can see their birth, their growth, their struggle for existence, their mode of nourishment by the absorption of living particles in the fluid by which they are surrounded, and, when old and shrunken, we can witness their final engulfment by the wandering cells of the body. To one of those cells, ignorant of the existence of that greater being of which it formed a tiny part, life would seem to be a meaningless struggle, a coming out of nothing and a departure into nothing. Only to us who are aware of the greater organism of which the cell is a part has the drama of its life and death any meaning. We are in a similar position to the cells whose birth and death and interesting struggles we have witnessed on the cinema screen. Our birth and death are mysteries which can only be solved by a knowledge of that greater being of which we form a tiny part.

As in life one part of a man ceases to grow before another, so in death does one tissue of the body die before another; in other words, the death of the body proceeds by stages. There is a longevity of the different tissues as well as a longevity of the whole organism. According to Ischlondsky the cells which have the power to survive longest are those which make up the central nervous system. It is interesting to note that the highest constituent of the body as well as the most evolved of the animals forming part of organic life, mankind, is one of the longest lived. As the brain cells are the most intelligent and the longest lived of all the cells of the body, so are men the most intelligent and among the longest lived of animals. Actually there are certain cells in the body which may be said never to die, namely the germinal cells which at an early stage of development are set aside for the purposes of reproduction. These immortal elements in us continue to live in our children when the rest of the body has perished. The germinal cells may be looked upon as forming an unbroken living chain which stretches from the present back to the dawn of life upon this planet. But only those germinal cells in us which have achieved their destiny and live in our children are immortal, and the rest of our physical being must die, not *en masse* but gradually and by stages.

The progressive death of the body is best illustrated by describing what sometimes happens when a patient collapses during a serious operation. It must be pointed out that this is of very rare occurrence at the present day and may only have happened two or three times in a surgeon's whole professional lifetime. When such a catastrophe does happen the patient's breathing suddenly stops, his heart ceases to beat, colour disappears from his lips, his pupils dilate, and, to all appearances, the patient has died. By means of heroic methods of resuscitation, the giving of oxygen, strychnine injections, heart massage and artificial respiration, the patient may revive, in the sense that the machinery of life is restarted; the pulse is felt again, the colour returns to the lips, and respiration is resumed. On being returned to the ward, the improvement may continue and the patient may sometimes even begin to take nourishment. But in spite of this dramatic revival, death generally occurs twenty-four to forty-eight hours later without the patient having recovered full consciousness. Total death has occurred because, in spite of the apparent recovery, local death of the brain has already taken place. Stronger tissues revived, and the patient appeared to have recovered, but actually he died on the operating table, when the vital centres in the brain, deprived of all fresh blood, were damaged beyond hope of repair. Occasionally such patients do recover, but this probably means that the circulation through the brain has never entirely ceased. Some fifteen years ago an interview with a patient who had recovered from a collapse on the operating table was published in a daily paper. He had little memory of what had happened beyond the memory that he had been sublimely happy and then, with much pain and suffering, had been dragged back to life. He had no complaints against the nurses and doctors who had only done their duty, but felt that they had deprived him of a peace which he had never before possessed. In view of the connection already made between survival and growth, it is interesting to note that the brain has the lowest capacity for growth of all the tissues of the body. It is generally supposed that nerve cells are incapable of reproducing themselves, and yet in the opinion of Ischlondsky they are potentially the longest lived. Fortunately we have been provided at birth with such a vast store of these nerve cells that they are sufficient for the rest of our lives. This incapacity for growth of nerve cells may at first sight appear to be incompatible with the statement previously made that growth was a sign of youth. It must be remembered, however, that the statement was made in connection with multicellular organisms. The inability of nerve cells to reproduce themselves probably supplies the reason for the brain being the first organ of the body to die. Such tissues as the hair and nails provide a striking contrast to it. These structures are endowed with a strong capacity for growth and are amongst the last of the tissues to die; it is well known that the beard continues to grow several hours after the rest of the body has died.

Our attitude to death tends to change at different periods of our lives, and Metchnikoff believes that a man develops, in the course of years, what he calls a natural instinct for death. As a tired man longs for sleep, so does one who has become old and infirm look forward to the enigmatic sleep of death. I do not believe that this philosophical view of death is developed by the majority of men, but I agree that it may be an attitude which is reached by certain individuals. So many amongst the old resent the thought of dying that I find it difficult to postulate the existence of a natural instinct for death. Charles Renovier, a French philosopher, who died at the age of 88, wrote as follows:

> I know that I am going to die, but I cannot *persuade* myself that I am going to die. It is not the philosopher in me that protests. The philosopher does not fear death; it is the *old man*. The old man has not the courage to submit to the inevitable.

There are many who, like Renovier, have not the courage to submit to the inevitable. Leopardi, the Italian poet, was haunted all his life by the idea of death, and protested angrily against it.

> Why alas, after the sad voyage of life, do you not make the arrival joyful? This certain end, this end which is in our souls all our lives, which alone can smooth out troubles, why do you drape it in black and surround it with mournful shades? Why do you make the harbour more terrible than the open seas?

But Leopardi is wrong, for it is man who makes death seem terrible, and who solemnizes his departure with black drapery and funeral rites. 'Pompa mortis magis terret quam mors ipsa.' (BACON.)

It is interesting to note the different attitudes to death of various people. In times of peace and in the highly civilized West, death is unobtrusive. The quiet and efficient undertakers carry out their work with discretion, and we seldom see anything which can shock our sensibilities. But in war, death's handiwork can no longer be hidden, and the soldier is continually reminded of the fate which awaits all mankind. In a certain communication trench leading to a particularly active part of the line, during the last War, there hung a grim *memento mori*. A corpse had been built into the walls of the parapet, and a gaunt arm, still encased in its tattered sleeve, had worked to the surface. It was impossible to avoid seeing that bony hand, which obtruded into the passage and seemed to beckon to us as we passed that way. At night the flickering of the star-shells imparted to it an illusion of movement and rendered it still more macabre. A few of the men deliberately looked the other way as they passed, and pretended that they had not noticed it, but the great majority made the withered hand a subject for merriment. 'How are you feeling to-night, old flick?' one would ask. 'Taking it easy, aren't you?' Another, bolder than the rest, shook hands affably, and then the whole line would break out into laughter. To see death as it was, to realize that at any moment their own warm bodies might join company with that cold hand was too difficult, and tacitly they had agreed to convert what was intolerable into a joke. It is a defence mechanism which is not uncommonly employed.

Our horror of death to some extent comes from the error of identifying the person with the physical body, and there was an element of sanity in these soldiers' attitude to an unknown companion's body. For them, that which had been left behind was no longer a man, but only something he had discarded. If we could accept it as a law of nature that our bodies come from organic life, and are returned to organic life in order that their elements may be used again, death would lose some of its horror. We have been lent the use of a body for a limited period, and cannot expect immortality of what is essentially mortal. Those who watch the final stages of natural death, the hard-drawn breath, the convulsive movements, should remember that the person they have loved has departed, and that these distressing struggles are nothing but the unconscious reflexes of the discarded body.

That fascinating old Chinese sage, Chuang Tzu, knew that the enigma of death was insoluble; but he was as ready to believe that its purpose was beneficial as that it was harmful.

> How do I know [he wrote] that love of life is not a delusion after all? How do I know but that he who dreads to die is as a child who has lost the way and cannot find his home?
> The lady Li Chi was the daughter of Ai Fêng. When the Duke of Chin first got her, she wept until the bosom of her dress was drenched with tears. But when she came to the royal residence, and lived with the Duke, and ate rich food, she repented of having wept. How then do I know but that the dead repent of having previously clung to life?
> Those who dream of the banquet wake to lamentation and sorrow. Those who dream of lamentation and sorrow wake to join the hunt. While they dream, they do not know that they dream. Some will even interpret the very dream they are dreaming: and only when they awake do they know it was a dream. By and by comes the Great Awakening, and then we find out that this life is really a great dream. Fools think they are awake now, and flatter themselves they know if they are really princes or peasants. Confucius and you are both dreams; and I who say you are dreams,—I am but a dream myself. This is a paradox. To-morrow a sage may arise to explain it; but that to-morrow will not be until ten thousand generations have gone by. (CHUANG TZU: Translation of Professor H. A. Giles.)

Chuang Tzu is not alone in picturing life as a dream from which the dreamer could awake perhaps in this life, perhaps in another. And he used these words deliberately and not in any figurative sense.

But whether we look upon death as the end, as did Leopardi and Aristotle, or agree with Chuang Tzu that it may be the moment of awakening from a dream, we are bound to come to the conclusion that death is a necessary corollary to life. It is impossible to visualize a world of the nature of ours from which death had been banished. It would be a world in which no beneficent limit was placed on suffering, a world filled with the maimed and the broken, a world impossible for the young, a world stagnant with worn-out traditions and incapable of progress. Actually everyone realizes this, and it is chiefly because his own and his loved ones' individualities must disappear that death seems terrible. Socrates, the wisest of all the Greeks, uttered these words:

> No one knows what death is, and whether it be not the greatest of all good things to man. Nevertheless it is feared as though it were the supreme evil.

And again after drinking his potion of hemlock:

> Wherefore be of good cheer about death and know for certainty that no evil can happen to a good man either in this life or after death. He and his own are not neglected by the gods nor has my own approaching end happened by mere chance. The hour of my departure has arrived and we go our ways — I to die and you to live. Which is better, God only knows.

There is a similarity in the attitude of all the great sages to the subject of death, a community of feeling which bridges the centuries and differences of clime and culture. A story is told of Chuang Tzu that

> when his wife died, Hueitse went to express his condolence but found Chuang Tzu squatting on the ground and singing a song, beating time by striking an earthen basin: 'Why, this woman has lived with you and borne you children. At the worst, you might refrain from weeping when her old body dies. Is it rather too much that you should beat the basin and sing?'
>
> And Chuang Tzu replied, 'You are mistaken. When she first died, I could not also help feeling sad and moved, but I reflected that in the beginning she had no life, she had no bodily shape; and not only no bodily shape, she had no ghost. Caught in this ever-changing flux of things, she became a ghost, the ghost became a body, and the body became alive. Now she has changed again and become dead, and by so doing she has joined the eternal procession of spring, summer, autumn and winter. Why should I make so much noise and wail and weep over her while her body lies quietly there in the big house? That would be a failure to understand the course of things. That is why I stopped crying.'

Despite nature's reputation for cruelty, the moment of death is generally freed from acute suffering and terror. Nature prepares her children for their departure, or, if it be an awakening, she rouses them from sleep gently. The gradual slowing down of the circulation deprives the brain of nourishment, so that the mind is no longer able

to register poignant impressions. As a rule the dying man is totally
unaware of what is happening to him. While his body is struggling for
breath, his spirit is already far away. It is only the spectators of the
body's fight for survival who feel that dying is difficult. What they
see is but the snapping of the last strands of the retaining ropes, and the
falling away of the props prior to the gliding of the craft into another
element.

But departure is not invariably preceded by a dimming of consciousness, and Sir James Crichton-Browne describes an interesting
death-bed phenomenon which he calls 'lightning before death'. This
term is taken from Shakespeare's lines:

> How oft have men when at the point of death
> Been merry, which their keepers call,
> The lightning before death?

He refers to a fleeting and dazzling flash of consciousness which
sometimes precedes its extinction, an ecstasy which makes all
things appear clear to the dying man. It is a moment of illumination, resembling that which is sometimes described by those who have
been rescued at the last moment from drowning. For the dying man
the clouds seem to part, giving him one fleeting glimpse of dazzling
truth. Even when 'lightning before death' does not attain the level of
a vision, it may be associated with the unleashing of powers that have
long been lying in abeyance. Crichton-Browne tells us, on Goethe's
authority, of an old man of the lower class who on his death-bed was
heard to recite passages from the Greek classics. It was afterwards
discovered that in his boyhood he had been compelled to commit to
memory passages of Greek, which had remained in his mind all his
life, only to be recalled at the moment of death. This revival of childhood memories at the moment of death would appear to be exceedingly
common. During the last world war I was working at a dressing-
station a short distance behind the lines, to which badly wounded men
of various nationalities were being brought for treatment. Over and
over again I heard dying men — and more particularly those of Latin
extraction — calling out for their mothers. As life was drawing to a
close, it seemed to be turning in the direction of its beginning, to the
far off days of childhood. Helpless, frightened and distressed, these

dying men had again become children who called out in the dark for that person who had always been the first to answer their cries. Death was closing the circle of their lives, the cycle of their time.

Medical men are called upon to fight for their patient's life, but sometimes death appears to them as an arch-benefactor instead of as an arch-enemy. Often it is the only possible solution for a hopeless situation. 'Thou alone, O Death,' wrote Aeschylus, 'art the healer of deadly ills', and Aeschylus must have seen much of death to have written those lines. Maeterlinck even protests against the efforts of medical men to drag back their dying patients to a life which may no longer contain anything of value to them. 'The dead', he writes, 'if they were to speak amongst themselves of a dying man whom the physician and surgeon were trying to save would say: "He is in danger of life"' (*The Hour-glass.*)

The same thought that death is the healer of ills for which there is no other satisfactory remedy was evidently in Sir Walter Raleigh's mind when he stood on the scaffold. It is recorded that before placing his neck on the block he examined the executioner's axe with a connoisseur's scrutiny. 'This is a sharp medicine', he said, 'but a sound cure for all diseases.' Raleigh was suffering at the time from malignant malarial fever, which, during the whole of his trial, had been so severe as to cause repeated attacks of shivering. He was a devoutly religious man with a strong faith in a future life, and may well have felt that death was the only medicine which would cure him of the ills which doctors had failed to relieve.

Many people are not so much frightened of death as of the act of dying. Those even who have no hope of personal survival may reconcile themselves to the thought of extinction and yet fear the process by which this is achieved. This is a strange anomaly, for whereas the fear of death itself can be excused on the grounds that it is instinctive and shared by the higher animals, in so far that they show fear in the presence of a dead body, the fear of the act of dying is acquired and essentially a human difficulty. It has been suggested that the fear of death is necessary to the preservation of the race, a fear which, according to Samuel Butler, is handed down by inherited memory. But the fear of the process of dying serves no useful purpose and is based on a misconception. It arises from the belief that the act of dying entails pain and mental suffering. This is an illusion which is the result of mistaking the convulsive movements of the body and its automatic struggles to maintain itself for voluntary movements made by a suffering man. What impresses those who have seen most of death, the doctors, is its gentleness, and I am continually being astonished by the smoothness of the ferrying across the Styx. Natural death entails a minimum of suffering, and even when the death is due to violence it is probably far less painful than those who witness it believe it to be. The consciousness of the dying man is dimmed and often he does not even realize that he is dying. The waters of Lethe have a soporific action on suffering in addition to effacing memory. When a man does realize that he is dying he seldom shows fear, or complains of any serious discomfort. John Hunter, one of the greatest figures in the history of English surgery, said on his death-bed: 'If I had strength enough to hold a pen I would write how easy and pleasant a thing it is to die.' These were his last words.

R. W. Mackenna endorses this view in his book, *The Adventure of Death*:

> It falls to most doctors to see much of death, and I have watched by the bedside of the dying of many classes and of all ages. I have seen the little silken thread on which a child's life hung — a life, so far as one could tell, of infinite potentialities for good — snap suddenly, leaving only a terrible sense of the mystery and inevitableness of it all; and I have fought death, and lost the battle, over the beds of young men and women in the first flush of maturity; and I have seen strong men and women cut down in their prime; and I have watched the old totter down the slope into twilight, and at the end fall asleep like children, and I say it with a due sense of the importance of this statement, that my experience has been that, however much men and women may, when in the full vigour of health fear death, when the hour approaches the fear is almost invariably stilled into gentleness, and they face the end with calmness and a serene mind.

The doctor and his patient are allies in the fight against death, and if they are to win they must co-operate to the fullest. But this unanimity of purpose does not always exist, for there are patients who, instead of struggling against illness and death, capitulate before the fight has been joined. We are told that there are natives of India, Africa and Australia who can voluntarily lie down and die. There are also patients who on entering a hospital or a nursing home lie down in bed and do likewise. They refuse to struggle, or if they struggle it is not against the common enemy, but against their allies, the doctors and nurses. They will accept none of the conditions which are necessary to their cure. If an operation be required, they fight with the anaesthetist, and even when the ether has at last taken effect they remain tense and rigid on the operating table. On regaining consciousness the fight is renewed, and only ends when the patient and his nurses are completely exhausted. No surgeon is wise to operate on a patient who is not prepared to co-operate to the best of his ability. He must not only outwardly agree to the carrying out of what may be deemed necessary, but inwardly acquiesce in his treatment. This type of refractory patient must not be confused with the patient who realizes that he is suffering from an incurable disease and quietly makes up his mind that a protracted fight for life is useless. It may be that according to his own way of thinking this is the most reasonable thing he can do in such circumstances.

The desirability, or not, of conferring on a doctor the right to end useless suffering has been much discussed of recent years, and it is not long since a euthanasia Bill was debated in Parliament. We have all been flung into this world without having been consulted whether we had a desire to be born and to grapple with life's problems or not. Have we the right to depart from it if living has become for us nothing but suffering? Here is a moral question, the answer to which must depend on our philosophy and our beliefs. What is the meaning of life? Is it, as some scientists would lead us to believe, a meaningless accident, or has it some deep unguessed significance? Whatever the answer may be to this question, and whether euthanasia be legalized or not, it is probable that a precise formulation of the circumstances in which it would be permitted, instead of making the work of medical men easier, would render it more difficult. The law is a clumsy mentor, as incapable of defining the responsibilities of a doctor to his patient as of regulating a relationship between friends. No doctor needs the assistance of a Justice of the Peace in deciding when it is necessary to relieve a hopeless sufferer. He prefers to consult his own conscience, and having consulted it. to do what he believes to be right. No patient need suffer if morphia be given in sufficient quantity and sufficiently often, and in the rare cases in which morphia fails, relief may be brought by dividing the path along which the pain messages travel. Doctors, like other citizens, must act in accordance with the laws of the land in which they live, but they do not look to these laws for guidance in their profession.

CHAPTER VIII

THE HEREAFTER

THE fact that a problem is insoluble does not preclude efforts to solve it, and man's inability to see beyond the grave does not prevent him from searching for some clue to the enigma of death. The hope of survival seems to be innate in mankind. Sir James Frazer states that 'men in all stages of ignorance and knowledge commonly believe that when they die some part of them does not perish', and the late Professor William McDougall gave it as his opinion that a belief in the doctrine of personal survival of death is essential to the moral welfare of any nation. The great majority of us have a strong desire to escape the extinction of all those thoughts and feelings, hopes and beliefs, the sum-total of which make up the individual man. And it is the individual that must continue to exist if we are to be satisfied. The survival of a consciousness stripped of all personal traits and memories would not content us. Yet if we look back on the few moments of pure emotion which we have enjoyed during our lives, moments of sheer delight amounting to almost ecstasy, we find that they are selfless. In the presence of a great truth and in a moment of heightened consciousness that poor dwarf, personal identity, shrinks into nothingness, and freed from the limitations it imposes upon us, we become part of some majestic whole. At those moments only that in us which transcends the personal would seem to be capable of surviving the dissolution of the body. If we have been conscious of the impermanence and futility of our personalities in those rare moments of understanding, how unlikely it is that they will outlive the dissolution of the body. I cannot believe that the Intelligence which planned the universe felt any necessity to preserve in perpetuity the poor tricks which distinguish me from my fellows. This 'self', which is entirely dependent on its environment, reacting with pleasure or pain to each change, cannot outlast the crumbling of the tissues; if this be all, it is doomed to perish.

When death comes near to man that which is mortal in him is scattered; that which is immortal and incorruptible withdraws intact. (SOCRATES.)

There is a passage in the *Mantic Al-Taqr* of Attar, the great Persian mystical poet, which describes this disappearance of the mortal element in man, the self which he clings to:

Whoever leaves this world behind him passes away from mortality, and when he has passed away from mortality, he attains to immortality. If thou findest thyself bewildered, O heart, pass over the bridge of Sirat[1] and the burning fires of Hell. Grieve not, for the flame from the oil in the lamp gives forth smoke black as an old crow, but when the oil has been consumed by that flame, it has ceased to exist as oil. If thou didst desire to reach this abode of immortality, and to attain to this exalted station, divest thyself first of self, then summon unto thyself a winged steed out of nothingness, to bear thee aloft. Clothe thyself with the garment of nothingness and drink the cup of self-annihilation. Cover thy breast with nothingness, and draw over thy head the robe of non-existence. Set thy foot in the stirrup of complete renunciation and, looking straight before thee, ride the steed of not-being to the place where nothing is. Thou wilt be lost again and again, yet go thy way in tranquillity, until at last thou shalt reach the world where thou art lost altogether to Self. (ATTAR: 'The Persian Mystics'. Wisdom of the East Series.)

McNeile Dixon, commenting on the almost universal desire for personal survival, writes:

That mortals should desire immortality and yet find it difficult to pass an afternoon — if you have a fancy for paradoxes, here is a pretty one. We contemplate eternity without horror, and find an hour of our society intolerable.

The paradox is less unresolvable than McNeile Dixon would have us believe. We attribute our discontent upon earth not to ourselves but to our circumstances, and in the heaven we create for ourselves circumstances are idealized. Adam, in Shaw's *Back to Methuselah*, voices the apprehensiveness felt by some people of the prospect of

---

[1] 'The bridge across Hell, which is thinner than a hair, and sharper than the edge of a knife.' (*Ibid.*)

eternal life, but it is an apprehensiveness of a life similar to life upon this earth carried on in perpetuity.

> If only there be an end some day, and yet no end. If only I can be relieved of the horror of having to endure myself for ever! If only the care of this terrible garden may pass on to some other gardener . . . If only the rest and sleep that enables me to bear it from day to day, could grow, after many days into an eternal rest, an eternal sleep, then I could face my days however long they may last. Only there must be some end. Some end; I am not strong enough to bear eternity.

Although there be no answer to this question of survival after death, it is interesting to review some of the attempts which have been made to solve the insoluble riddle.

It may be that the materialistic scientist is right and that death is the end of everything. So many of the scientist's statements have been found to be correct that his opinion on this all-important subject must be treated with respect. At the same time it may be pointed out that the idea of survival is fundamental in scientific thought. The scientist has found it necessary to accept the principle of the indestructibility of matter and energy, the concepts with which he is chiefly concerned. If he were to admit the existence of spirit, he would probably find it necessary also to accept the doctrine of its survival of death. It is to the scientist and not to the priest or the prophet that we now turn for guidance. We pride ourselves on having shed the superstition of our forefathers, who lived in a pre-scientific and what we consider to have been a less enlightened age, but there always exists the uncomfortable possibility that we have only exchanged one set of superstitions for another. Whilst our ancestors were credulous of priests, we may be harbouring a childish faith in scientists. Whether this be so or not, it is a fact that when we demand of the scientist a ruling on the subject of survival after death, we are asking him to adjudicate outside his legitimate sphere. The scientist deals with matter and with knowledge which is gained through the medium of the special senses. Consciousness cannot be observed, weighed or measured, and it is to the philosopher and the man of religion that we must go for an answer to the enigma of death. Whilst the scientist talks the language of matter, the philosopher and the mystic, whether Christian, Hindu, Buddhist or

Sufi, talks the language of the spirit. Though their words are sometimes difficult to understand, they alone are capable of dealing with this subject.

Many of the guesses that have been made about the future life are extremely naïve, and are clear examples of wish-fulfilment. The warriors of the North created for their dead a gargantuan Valhalla, where the mead was strong and the company uproarious. To the roystering Vikings of Scandinavia the future life took the form of a prolonged wassail. For such a hunting people as the North American Indians there lay beyond the tomb a Happy Hunting Ground, and for the pleasure-loving, sensuous Mohammedan, gaudy palaces peopled by almond-eyed houris. All these ideas of an existence beyond the grave have this in common, that they visualize life as continuing much as it was lived upon earth, but under idealized conditions. This method of creating a glorified earthly existence still survives amongst us, and is apparent in spiritualistic thought. Many spiritualists envisage the dead as living in some ghostly suburbia, which provides the same pleasures of whisky and cigars for the men, and tea and talk for the women. In nebulous surroundings the dead beguile the tedium of eternity with the time-killing devices which proved so helpful on earth. The crudity of the spiritualist's vision is strictly in keeping with the subconscious ideals of the medium who is acting as its interpreter. Since we build our heavens out of the material in our minds, it would be altogether surprising if, from the brain of an ill-educated medium, were evolved a vision of the future on the grand scale of Dante's *Divina Comedia*.

This does not necessarily imply that all the phenomena of the séance can be summarily dismissed as being the result of deliberate fraud, or of the working of the subconscious mind. For more than half a century critical, as well as credulous, investigators have been engaged in psychical research. An examination of the *Proceedings of the Society for Psychical Research* shows that every effort has been made to carry out its investigations in a scientific spirit. Those who have taken part in the research have been fully alive to the tricks which may be played on us by the more submerged parts of the mind, and to the possible intervention of telepathy. When the available evidence has been carefully sifted and critically examined, there still remains a residuum for which no explanation can be found. The spiritualists themselves accept this as a definite proof of survival after death. This, however, is neither the only, nor, on the whole, the most likely explanation of it. What the inexplicable phenomena of the séance suggests is that the minds of even ordinary men possess certain latent powers and unknown capacities of apprehension not under 'their control, but which sometimes come into action accidentally. Because the knowledge within the range of these latent faculties is knowledge which we do not ordinarily possess, it is believed to come from an outside source. It is natural that the spiritualists who above all are anxious to find support for personal survival after death should believe this source to be a departed spirit. The error lies not in the claim that inexplicable happenings sometimes occur but in the explanation of these happenings. Writing of the four more important and well-attested phenomena of the séance, telepathy, clairvoyance, precognition and retrocognition, G. N. M. Tyrrell states that no theory which has yet been put forward succeeds in keeping 'psychic phenomena within the orbit of the familiar and known'. He complains that because the psychic manifestations recorded by the Society for Psychical Research are so revolutionary that they would necessitate a reconstruction of their ideology, scientists dismiss them as unproven without bothering to examine whether this be the case or not:

> When we look deeply into the nature of human personality, we find that vistas of the self are hidden behind the scenes, possessing powers and qualities which science is unable to define, or bring into line with other knowledge by its superficial methods . . . It overturns the complacency of successful science, which has been dealing with the surface-appearance of things based on the findings of the senses.

In giving his own opinion of the problem of survival after death Tyrrell writes:

> What psychical research suggests is that the complex personality is resolved at death. This resolution is not so much a process of a 'thing' coming to an end, as of a group-complex reshaping, or changing its internal relations. It need not destroy the intrinsic character of the constituents; in particular, it need not destroy the principle of the dominant 'I' . . . The idea would be more easily expressed by saying that selfhood *transcends* the conditions of the

present world in some non-temporal way — Time, at any rate as we understand it, being one of the conditions of the present highly special world accompanying one special grouping of the personality. (*Science and Psychical Phenomena.*)

In the East the view which is most widely held is that the spirit after death reincarnates in a new body. 'As a man discards his threadbare robes and puts on new, so the Spirit throws off its worn-out bodies and takes fresh ones' (*Bhagavad-gita*). The idea of the transmigration of the soul is the oldest of all attempts to solve the riddle of life and death. From Vedic literature it passed into Buddhism to reappear in Greece in the beliefs of the Orphici and the Pythagoreans. The doctrine of metempsychosis undoubtedly influenced the writings of Pindar, Empedocles and Plato, and was probably well known in Judea at the time of Christ. It is difficult otherwise to explain the question put to Christ, 'Master, who sinned, this man or his parents that he was *born* blind?' The form in which the idea of the transmigration of the soul is presented is sometimes crude and fanciful, but it is entirely compatible with philosophical thought, as was freely admitted by Schopenhauer: 'Never has a myth and never will a myth be more closely connected with philosophical truth, which is difficult to grasp, than the primeval doctrine professed by a most noble and ancient race [The Hindus].'

It must indeed be admitted that the Hindu teaching is in this matter more logical than that of the Christian Church, for if the soul be immortal it must be without beginning as well as without end. Baron Palmstierna, in a recent book (*Towards a Single Faith*), advances the view that Christ, His followers, and such early Christian writers as Origen, actually took the pre-existence of the soul for granted, but that the theory of the 'pilgrim soul' was excluded from Church teaching at the time of St. Athanasius and the Council of Nicaea. This may well be so, for the year of the Council of Nicaea was undoubtedly one of the most disastrous in the history of the Christian Church. The idea of reincarnation is closely linked with another Eastern doctrine, the doctrine of Karma. To the Hindu, justice is impersonal and automatic, and it is not dependent on the whim of a deity. As a man sows in one life, so shall he reap in another; if he meets with misfortune in his present existence, this is the direct result of past errors and misdeeds which he now has a chance to expiate by acceptance and right effort. We make a mistake when we describe this attitude of the Hindu as being negative and fatalistic. The Hindu is strictly scientific in his outlook, for he looks upon all psychic experiences as being determined by the law of cause and effect. Reincarnation is a necessary complement to the doctrine of Karma, for it would be difficult to suppose that a man could reach that stage of enlightenment and full development of faculties latent in him, which the Hindu believes to be the goal towards which humanity is striving in the short span of one lifetime. Therefore the Hindu believes that the pilgrim soul has undergone a long succession of rebirths in lower forms of life upon the earth before it has reached the level of human incarnation. And having evolved as far as humanity, it must continue the round of rebirths until the higher possibilities latent in man have been fully developed. Only then is the spirit liberated from the ceaseless round of birth and rebirth to exist on some higher level of being.

According to one Tibetan teaching a short period between two incarnations is passed by the spirit in an intermediate state. This is the doctrine of the 'Bardo', a doctrine which Madame David-Neel tells us is regarded by Tibetan scholars as being 'the exoteric expression of esoteric theories concerning death'. Deprived after death of all new sense-impressions, the discarnate consciousness ruminates on all the ideas which have previously been accumulated. 'The visions which it sees, which disconcert, or stupefy, or delight, or terrify it, are nothing but subjective images, projected by itself, and illustrating its own beliefs, its passions, and, in general, all the conduct of the mind of the deceased.' (*Buddhism*, by Alexandra David-Neel.) In order to liberate itself from this immediate state of existence the consciousness must realize the fundamental unreality of the scenes which it is witnessing. It must know that it is a mirage, an objectivation of thoughts, a hallucination produced by the longings and passions of its past life. Then only can it escape from the environment which its existence on earth has created for it, and leaving the Bardo return to another circle of life.

CHAPTER IX

THE CIRCLE OF RECURRENCE

WIDELY though the ideas of survival reviewed in the last chapter may differ they all have this in common, that they regard time as a line along which we are travelling, from the past to the present, and from the present to the future. The enigma of birth and death is bound up with our understanding of time, and time is a problem which has taxed the ingenuity of philosophers for thousands of years. It is impossible to discuss survival without reference to our understanding of time, and intricate though the subject may be, something must be said about it. For our present purposes it will be sufficient to consider time from the standpoint of dimensions. We live in a four-dimensional world, three dimensions of which we call space, and a fourth which we place in a separate category and call time. This fourth dimension of time appears utterly different in quality to the three dimensions of space—length, height and breadth, and is experienced as a succession of states, a sequence of fleeting moments. The 'now' disappears in a flash into the past, giving place to a new 'now', drawn from what, up till then, was the future. We live poised on the crumbling edge of the moment, the past existing for us as a memory, the future as a hope. So fundamentally different does this dimension of time appear to be from length, height and breadth, that, when the mathematicians stated that the separation our minds had made was only useful within a certain scale, and that when dealing with astronomical phenomena we must substitute a space-time continuum, we were bewildered. It seemed ridiculous to fuse into a featureless whole the old familiar entities of space and time. And for all practical purposes it is ridiculous to do so. We have learnt to perceive length, height and breadth as one thing, and the series of changes which we call time as another, and this arrangement serves our purposes admirably. If mathematicians and physicists find the convention unsatisfactory when studying the behaviour of the electron, or the movements of the heavenly bodies, it is their own affair. A space-time continuum may suit the mathematician and the scientist, but personally we prefer to retain the familiar division into space and time. We continue therefore to think of ourselves as existing in space and persisting in time. But in discussing such problems as birth and death, we are leaving the familiar world of everyday life and are groping after ideas which are far more elusive than an electron, and more difficult to comprehend than a magnetic field. Modes of thought which are justified on the grounds that they have proved sufficient for everyday purposes can no longer be retained. Having embarked upon a search for an answer to the question: Do we survive after death? we must equip ourselves with all that is necessary for conducting such a difficult inquiry. Amongst other changes that we may have to make is the substitution of a new concept for our familiar, and more limited, conception of time. We can best understand what the mathematician means when he states that our conception of time is illusory by the use of a parable.

Flatland: A Romance of Many Dimensions, written under the pseudonym of 'A Square' (by E. A. Abbott), provides us with a brilliant analogy of our own position with regard to time. The author describes the life of certain flat beings, who live in a two-dimensional world, and are utterly incapable of appreciating more than the two dimensions of length and breadth. The third dimension of height is beyond their powers of comprehension. A certain Flatlander, 'A Square', who is supposed to be the author of the book, receives a revelation. He is visited by a higher three-dimensional being, a Sphere. Because this mysterious visitor can move in the third dimension, he has the power to materialize within the Flatlander's house in the form of a widening circle. At first the circle is seen only as a line, but by walking round it the Flatlander realizes that the strange apparition is actually a circle. When the visitor makes movements at right angles to the two-dimensional world, strange things seem to be happening, the circle growing larger or smaller and eventually disappearing altogether. This is because only that section of the Sphere which coincides with his own plane is visible to the Flatlander, those parts of the Sphere which lie above and below it being beyond his ken. The changes in the circle are revealed to the Flatlander as a sequence of changes in time. The Sphere attempts to explain to the Flatlander that these changes co-exist in another dimension, but as his explanation proves unavailing, he decides to give the incredulous Flatlander an actual experience of the third dimension. Seizing him, he drags him out of his two dimensional plane into a higher world, that of three dimensions, returning him to his own more limited world after he has learnt his lesson. The story closes on a sombre note. The Flatlander, converted by his mystical experience to the idea of the third dimension, attempts to teach the new doctrine to his fellow-citizens. The only result is that he is thrown into prison charged with the offence of expounding heretical views on the nature of reality.

The analogy of 'Flatland' may be applied to our three-dimensional Spaceland. Like the Flatlanders, we, the Spacelanders, find it impossible to comprehend an additional dimension otherwise than as a sequence of changes in time. Whatever the mathematicians may tell us, we interpret our experiences in this dimension as a movement in time, from past, through present to future. Yet, to a consciousness higher than our own, the dimension revealed to us only in sequence might appear no different in kind from the three dimensions of space. This higher intelligence would be able to view the whole life pattern of this earth, and of ourselves, unravelled in space, the past not surviving merely as history, and the future existing only as a theme for prophecy, but past, present and future would be viewed extended in another dimension. This higher being would understand the difficulty encountered by the earth's inhabitants when they attempted to think of the fourth dimension. They would think that they were in constant movement and being carried along by a flowing river of time. They would be convinced that only the 'now' existed, that the past had perished, and that the future had not yet been created. To people of such limited comprehension the idea of past, present and future coexisting would seem to be utterly fantastic. They were like flies which crawled over the face of a statue and believed that each new feature they discovered had only just come into existence. The higher being might well feel some pity for these naïve little creatures, who, in spite of their limited perception, were attempting to solve the problem of survival after death by the crude method of extending the duration of their imaginary movement indefinitely into space. They were comforting themselves with a picture of plunging into a gloomy tunnel of death and then emerging into the sunshine of some new and highly idealized country. Their only conception of eternity was as of an everlasting journey along a never-ending line, a line which had a beginning but no end. Small wonder that the Spacelanders found their efforts to understand birth and death beset with insuperable difficulties. Was it the child, the youth, the middle-aged or the senile man whom they believed to be travelling after death along the long line of eternity? And did this tireless traveller grow older and older, or did he remain the same whilst all around him changed? Of this nature would be the thoughts of a greater intelligence who witnessed our efforts to solve a question which, for us, is insoluble.

There are two theories of survival which do not suffer from the objection of being based on an over-simplified view of time. The first, which need not long detain us, is that suggested by J. W. Dunne. Dunne started his investigations in order to throw light on what he had frequently observed, namely, that he had dreamt of future events. On talking to his friends and acquaintances he found that many of them, although they made no claim to be clairvoyant, had had similar experiences. Having confirmed these observations to the best of his ability he developed a theory which is set forth in his two books, *An Experiment with Time* and *The Serial Universe*. Briefly stated Dunne's explanation of precognition is that in all of us are different 'I's', or Observers, which exist and move in different dimensions of time. When we are asleep an Observer other than that which is associated with our waking moments may view events which lie farther along the line of past, present and future, and may reproduce them in dreams. We are not concerned here with the correctness or the incorrectness of Dunne's explanation of precognition, and there are many inconsistencies and ambiguities in his exposition of it, but rather with its bearing on the question of survival. At the beginning of his research he imagined that his belief in precognition would lead him to a deterministic philosophy and a disbelief in the possibility of survival after death. Instead he found himself driven to believe in 'the existence of an individual soul whose immortality, being in other dimensions of time, does not clash with the obvious ending of the individual'.

The second theory of survival based on a more philosophical view of time is the idea of Eternal Recurrence. This theory, which is generally associated with the name of Nietzsche, has recently been commented upon and developed by P. D. Ouspensky. Because Nietzsche reached this idea through his emotions and wrote of it as a poet rather than as a philosopher, it is to Ouspensky's work, *A New Model of the Universe*, that we must turn for a clear account of eternal recurrence. It is true that Nietzsche attempted to rationalize the idea which he had conceived as a poet, but his explanation is based on faulty premises. He argued that by the continued action of the same forces in the universe a similar earth would be created in which the same phenomena would be eventually reproduced.[1] Amongst these phenomena will be the same people who will live the same lives down to the smallest detail. But as Ouspensky points out Nietzsche failed to see that with each increase in the number of factors concerned there is an enormous increase in the number of combinations of them that are possible. With such a large number of factors as those which had determined our existence, the probability of an identical combination of them can be expressed as zero. No attempt will be made to summarize here Ouspensky's exposition of the idea of eternal recurrence. All that need be said is that according to this theory the 'soul' does not reincarnate as another being but is born again to repeat in every detail the previous cycle of life. Each new cycle begins in exactly the same manner as did the previous one, the moment of birth coinciding with the moment of death. Life is lived under precisely similar conditions and every event of the previous cycle is repeated in detail. With each repetition individual tendencies, both good and bad, tend to become strengthened. Although the idea of recurrence cannot be proved by direct observation, it is, in Ouspensky's opinion, in harmony with our knowledge of the nature of time. Time, according to this writer, has three dimensions, only one of which we can discern, the line along which we appear to be travelling, from the past to the present and from the present to the future. Our ordinary conception of life is of progress along a *straight* line, but dimensions of time, like those of space, are not really straight, but *curved*. This being so, man moves in a circle, approaching, as he grows older, the point in the circle at which he is reborn. He repeats and repeats the circle of his life in eternity,

[1] Compare Herodotus: 'Let time be lavished and all that is possible will come to pass.'

which is not a line indefinitely prolonged, but a circle which lies in the second dimension of time.

> One life ends and another begins. One time ends and another begins. Death is really a return to the beginning.

In addition to the intellectual arguments which may be advanced in favour of the idea of recurrence, there exists certain supporting evidence of an emotional character.

Many people at some moment of their lives have been overwhelmed by the feeling that 'all this has happened before'. They have a strong conviction that on some previous vaguely remembered occasion they have been in the same situation, doing the same thing and saying the same words to the same people. A striking example of this experience can be found in the *Journal* of Sir Walter Scott, an example which is of greater value because of the fact that Scott was not the type of man to claim or desire any psychic powers. Under the heading of February 17th, 1828, he writes:

> I cannot, I am sure, tell if it is worth marking down, that yesterday at dinnertime I was strangely haunted by what I would call the sense of pre-existence — videlicet, a confused idea that nothing that passed was said for the first time, that the same topics had been discussed, and the same persons stated the same opinions on the same subjects. It is true there might have been some ground for recollection, considering that three at least of the company were old friends, and kept much company together: that is, Justice Clerk, Abercrombie and I. But the sensation was so strong as to resemble what is called a 'mirage' in the desert, or a calenture on board ship, when lakes are seen in the desert and sylvan landscapes in the sea. It was very distressing yesterday, and brought to my mind the fancies of Bishop Berkeley about an ideal world. There was a vile sense of want of reality in all I did and said. It made me gloomy and out of spirits, though I flatter myself it was not observed. The bodily feeling which most resembles this unpleasing hallucination is the giddy state which follows profuse bleeding, when one feels as if walking on feather beds and could not find a secure footing. I think the stomach has something to do with it. I drank several glasses of wine, but these only augmented the disorder. I did not find the 'in vino veritas' of the

philosophers. Something of this insane feeling remains to-day, but a trifle only.

Scientists have offered a variety of explanations of this feeling of an experience having happened before. Medical men are by training disposed to regard all unusual psychic phenomena as being pathological, and Sir William Gower considered the phenomenon of the 'déjà vu' to be a variety of minor epilepsy. Sir James Crichton-Browne includes it in the category of 'dreamy mental states'. Others have explained the experience by the memory of a dream which approximated to the actual experience. Dunne is of the opinion that in dreams we may actually live through moments which in reality await us in the future, and he would probably regard this phenomenon as a confirmation of his theory. Another explanation of this feeling of recurrence is that it is due to a similarity, but not to an identity, of circumstances. This seems to be the most reasonable of the scientific explanations, but it does not account for the intense feeling of conviction which accompanies this form of memory.

Bergson (*Mind-Energy*, translated by H. Wildon Carr) has reviewed the literature of this phenomenon in a paper entitled, 'Memory of the Present and False Recognition'. After dismissing as unsatisfactory the various theories which have been put forward by physiologists and psychologists, he suggests an explanation based on his own interpretation of the nature of perceptions and memories. According to Bergson every moment of our psychic life presents two aspects, that of perception and that of memory. Two images of an object are created in us simultaneously, the first as a direct perception, the second, a reflection of it in memory. It is as though we viewed an object in front of a mirror, perceiving it directly and at the same time its reflection. In ordinary states we are not conscious of this duplication of psychic processes, but in exceptional circumstances we may become aware of it. Because we associate memory with something which has existed in the past we are deluded into believing that this reduplication means that we have perceived the object before. But actually we have caught a glimpse of a memory that does not lie in the past but in the present.

Ouspensky gives many references to writings in which the idea of eternal recurrence appears. He is of the opinion that it existed in the teaching of Pythagoras and that it may have been implicit in some of the early Christian beliefs. But the most vivid emotional writing on this subject will be found in *Thus Spake Zarathustra*. The idea of eternal recurrence came to Nietzsche with such force that he has written:

> The moment in which I begot recurrence is immortal, for the sake of that moment alone, I will endure recurrence. (*The Twilight of the Idols.*)

The idea of eternal recurrence is developed in a conversation between Zarathustra and his Beasts. Zarathustra has just recovered from a blinding vision, so overwhelming that for a time it had seemingly deprived him of consciousness. He speaks to his companion Beasts as a prophet, recounting to them the nature of his vision, and the Beasts not only accept, but corroborate the truth of his message.

> All goeth, all returneth; eternally rolleth the wheel of Being. Being buildeth itself. All things separate, all things greet one another again; for ever the Ring of Being remaineth true to Itself.
>
> At each moment Being returneth; about every *Here* revolveth the ball *There*. The centre is everywhere. Curved is the pathway of eternity.

To these words of Zarathustra his beasts, the Serpent and the Eagle, reply:

> For thy beasts well know, O Zarathustra, what thou art and must become. Behold, thou art the Teacher of Eternal Recurrence — *that* is *thy* fate!
>
> Behold, we know what thou teachest; that all things recur eternally, and we ourselves with them, and that we have been infinite times already, and all things with us.

And Zarathustra answers:

> I come again, with this sun, with this earth, with this Eagle, with this Serpent — *not* to a new life, or to a better life, or to a similar life —

I come again eternally to this selfsame life, in greatest things and in least, that I may teach again the Eternal Recurrence of all things.

The theories of Eternal Recurrence and of Reincarnation both recognize the principle of causality, a man's actions in one cycle of existence being conditioned by his actions in a previous cycle. Either he rises, or he sinks, his evolution or degeneration being determined by his own efforts. This being so, his every action becomes of supreme importance to him, as it is not an isolated event, but an event which will bear fruit in innumerable cycles of existence. According to these theories we do not live in an evanescent 'now', but in a 'now' which is being continually reborn. It is not a fleeting life which we are shaping, but an eternal life.

Many may feel that such theories as these are fantastic and that they run counter to common sense. But so also do many scientific theories seem fantastic and contrary to common sense, and yet because of the prestige conferred upon them by their origin they are readily accepted. What could appear more nonsensical at first hearing than the modern physicist's description of matter? Our attempts to visualize the physicist's description of the apparently solid material which surrounds us, and of which we ourselves are made, leave our minds confused and bewildered. We inwardly protest, but because we are assured by the scientists that their theories are based on the latest observations, we tentatively accept their words. Whether we have understood these words or not, we have, at any rate, gained valuable insight into the limitations of thinking, an insight which should be of value to us at the present moment. If we are plunged into a state of confusion when trying to visualize the nature of matter, how can we expect to fare better when engaged on the infinitely more difficult task of unravelling the mystery of life and death? How humiliatingly small is the sum total of our knowledge, and how little do we really understand. With what a display of words do we tell ourselves nothing about the eternal mysteries. If someone were to return from the grave to teach us about death, we would not be able to grasp his message.

We stretch our minds to the breaking-point in our effort to encompass the meaning of death, and still it eludes us. Is it the end, or the beginning? And if the latter, the beginning of what? Is it the beginning of a new extra-corporeal living, or, as the theory of eternal recurrence would have it, the return to an identical cycle of existence? The intellect alone can never tell us, and our emotions, caught by the lure and the glitter of life, we cannot trust. Only the seers who have transcended the narrow limits of the self, and who have risen above teach us, the meaning of death. They can only teach us what is on the level of our understanding.

PART TWO

CHAPTER I

DOCTORS AND DOCTORING

So far we have been studying the problems with which a doctor is called upon to deal, at one time viewing from afar the great insoluble questions which eternally challenge us, the mystery of birth and death, and at other times returning to examine the smaller phenomena of the consulting-room. But the practice of medicine, and it is out of this that this book has grown, entails the activity of treatment, as well as that of diagnosis. A doctor must find a remedy for the troubles which a patient brings to him. However impotent he may feel himself to be to deal with his patient's trouble, some remedy must be prescribed, some wise suggestions offered, and the patient sent away, comforted and fortified by the knowledge that something has been done to ease his discomfort and ensure his recovery. It will be necessary, therefore, to narrow our view and study for the time being some of the medical aspects of the problems we have been examining.

Let it be confessed at the very beginning of this description of doctors and doctoring, that the art of treatment lags far behind the art of diagnosis. We are more likely to know what is wrong with our patients than to be able to cure them. This fact is generally recognized and it has been made the subject of many jokes; for example, Hilaire Belloc's description of a medical consultation:

> They answered as they took their fees,
> 'There is no cure for this disease'.

But fortunately, his inability to find a remedy for a particular illness does not render the medical man entirely useless. Even if a doctor cannot cure his patient of a cold, he can relieve him of the fear that his sore throat may be due to diphtheria. A sick man wants to know exactly what is wrong with him. Is his illness serious or not? Why has this happened to him? How long is the disease likely to last? If a name can be attached to his disorder, even a freak name incomprehensible to the patient, if its nature is explained and reassurance given that he will be well again in a few days or weeks, a patient's mind is set at rest, and his illness may then become of secondary importance to him. What we understand and believe we can explain has lost half its terror for us, for it is the mysterious and the inexplicable which we most fear. This is particularly true of illness, and even if a doctor is unable to attach a name to a vague malady, or is doubtful in his own mind precisely why his patient has contracted it, he will generally be wiser to attach to it a label, and specify a cause.

Fortunately the doctor is helped in treatment by an ally wiser and infinitely better equipped than himself for bringing about a cure. 'Je le pensay, et Dieu le guérit', wrote Ambroise Paré, one of the most original men who ever practised medicine. Paré lived in a religious age when doctors believed in the existence of a beneficent purpose in the universe, and in the watchfulness of a Personal Deity, whom all creation served, and he was not afraid to invoke His name. Since the days of Ambroise Paré scientists have struggled hard to dethrone the Deity, and to substitute for Him a First Cause and a welter of inter-acting forces, and as Aldous Huxley has warned us, God is 'one of the words which the Mrs. Grundys of the intellect find particularly shocking'. Paré's medical successors are therefore shy of mentioning the Deity in connection with their work, and prefer to give the credit for the healing of wounds to a force which they refer to as the 'vis medicatrix naturae'. But nature, as we have seen, is far from being benevolent in her dealings with man, for to nature man is merely a constituent of organic life and of no particular consequence to her. It is not to nature, but to the patient's body, that credit should be given for the healing of wounds and recovery from disease. And, unlike nature, the patient's body has a keen interest in his physical welfare. The body has not only a strong will to live, but is also possessed of great cunning in achieving its ends. 'Who hath put wisdom in the inward parts? (Job xxxviii, 36).

The body has learnt its lesson in a hard school from which it has graduated with honours. Life from its first appearance on this planet has had to struggle tooth and nail in order to maintain its precarious hold upon the earth, and has survived only by virtue of its tenacity and dexterity in defending itself from the hostile forces by which it is surrounded. Bergson chose his words carefully when he referred to this great force of living as the 'élan vital'. The system of equilibrium which we call life has victoriously defied the massed forces of the material world, and frail though it may seem to be, it is imbued with unexpected strength. Whatever life may mean to man's intellect and his emotions, for his body it is a priceless gift from which it will never willingly be parted. Men have often sacrificed their existence for great or trivial causes, but their bodies have invariably protested against such wanton behaviour. Never did a body submit willingly to martyrdom. We are told that at a critical stage of a battle Frederick the Great galloped up to some troops which were retreating before superior forces of the enemy, shouting: 'Scoundrels, would you wish to live for ever! Advance!' History does not record how the soldiers responded to this appeal to their emotions. For it was to their emotions only that their monarch was speaking. If their bodies had answered the imperial exhortation the response would have been unanimous. 'Yes, Sire. We would live for ever. We would live to the last hard-drawn breath, to the final faint flicker of our hearts. We care not a groat for your high-sounding phrases, your honour and your glory.'

Were it not for the courage and cunning of the patient's body, devoting all its energies to a single end, the doctor would be but a poor figure of fun. Often his sole work is to hold, as it were, a watching brief, and to stand at the patient's bedside and ensure that nothing is done which will hamper the recuperative powers of his patient's constitution. Hippocrates was well aware of the limited rôle played by the doctor when he laid down the guiding principle that if a physician could do no good, he must make certain that he did no harm. The father of medicine spoke with his customary wisdom, for inaction in a crisis may sometimes be more difficult than action, and there are doctors who are sorely tempted to cover up their impotence with a display of energy. It was with some justification that a cynic wrote: 'Young physicians kill their patients, whilst old ones let them die.'

Doctors have the help of their patients' body and in many cases of their emotions also. Faith is a worker of miracles, not only through the mediumship of the spiritual healer, but also through that of the medical man. If a doctor can inspire confidence in his patient, and enable him to substitute a quiet optimism for panic, he will have done much to create conditions favourable to recovery. Herein lies the explanation of the excellent results often obtained by charlatans and dealers in magical nostrums. Fear, as we have seen, has physical repercussions on the body, and faith is its appropriate antidote, whether it be faith in the remedies prescribed, or faith in the prescriber. Most sick people are either mildly perturbed, or actually frightened by the mysterious power which holds them in its grip. They are in need of reassurance and comfort, and the physician who can impart these has already achieved much.

The most successful physician I have ever met was a Dr. Luis Guemes, who practised in Buenos Aires. He started seeing patients at his house at eight in the evening, and continued without interruption until three next morning. Each patient on his arrival in the crowded waiting-room received a card with a number, and the doctor's butler made a considerable income in dealing these out. When Guemes appeared at the door of his consulting-room on the first floor, bidding a patient good-bye, there was a rush of female patients up the stairs in the hope of touching him, for to many he seemed to be possessed of super-natural powers. Patients, relatives and practitioners who had called him into consultation left his presence with the deep conviction that he had conferred some lasting benefit on them. The secret of his outstanding success was his genius to dispense hope. Even if the patient died within an hour oi his departure, the relatives exclaimed: 'I shall never forget Dr. Guemes. He was the only doctor who gave us any hope.' Dr. Guemes was a very great physician, of exceptional clinical ability, and with a rare understanding of human nature.

Although such a striking instance of belief in the personal magic of a physician is rare, it exists very commonly in a much lesser degree. There is something of the child in most sick adults, a stirring in them of old ideas about magic, and an awakening of a desire for the performance of miracles. Patients do not look for an ordinary human being like themselves to cure them, but for a superior being possessing the powers of a wizard. If their ordinary medical attendant cannot fill this rôle, they will seek out somebody who can, a quack, a dealer in strange remedies, a doctor with a foreign name, a bone-setter, a healer without any medical qualification; or, if they have no imagination, merely a man living in Harley Street. Although my opinion cannot escape being prejudiced I am very doubtful whether books, written for the express purpose of exposing the futility of the medical profession, serve a useful purpose. If there be any better equipped for the task of dealing with disease than the doctors, then by all means let us expose the weaknesses and failings of the medical profession. But if there be no choice, if the doctors are our only resource, and if on the whole they have shown themselves to be more successful than the charlatans are, do not make their work still more difficult and ineffectual by depriving them of their most potent remedy, the faith and confidence of their patients. Because of the desire for wonder-working, few doctors make satisfactory medical advisers for their own relatives or intimate friends. I am doubtful whether even Mesmer would have achieved his remarkable cures had he remained amongst his own people, for a physician, like a prophet, has no honour in his own country.

It is not surprising that occasionally — and it is of rare occurrence — a medical man abuses the faith placed in him and utilizes for his own, rather than for his patients' profit, the power which this gives him. The descent from the employment of legitimate methods of suggestion to rank quackery is so gradual as to be almost imperceptible. This is well illustrated by the history of that brilliant and remarkable pioneer in psycho-therapy, Mesmer. Mesmer obtained so many cures by his method of treatment that the French Government appointed a special scientific committee to discover his secret. He cannot therefore be lightly dismissed as a charlatan. Yet in order to create the right emotional atmosphere for his treatment he made use of a great deal of mummery: strange lights played about the salon in which his patients were collected, sounds of soft music were heard coming from an adjoining room, and at the right moment Mesmer himself appeared, dressed in strange clothes. Mesmer was considered to be a quack by the majority of his medical contemporaries, but he was a sincere man and he made use of all this pantomime in order to secure favourable surroundings for treatment by suggestion. He used methods which were redolent of quackery, but what distinguished him from a charlatan was that whilst the latter works to further his own ends, Mesmer's main concern was his patients' cure.

In the preface to *The Doctor's Dilemma* Bernard Shaw proclaims that it is an illusion to believe that medicine is a science and that doctors are scientists; 'the rank and file of doctors are no more scientific than their tailors'. But Shaw is vociferously denying the validity of a claim which doctors would be the last to put forward. Medicine has gained immensely from its association with biology, chemistry and physics, but itself remains an art. There are so many gaps in a medical man's knowledge that he, like a tailor, must work empirically, and by the slow method of trial and error. If Shaw wishes to place us in the same category as tailors, he is at liberty to do so, for tailoring, like the practice of medicine, is not a science, but a blending of science and art. We make no claim to be scientists.

Modern civilized man has profoundly altered the conditions under which he lives, and by so doing has eliminated many of the illnesses from which his forefathers suffered. He has, at the same time, substituted for these others of his own making. The company promoter, who lives in a state of chronic anxiety, checkered by bouts of excitement, who eats three large meals a day, never walks when it can be avoided, stimulates his flagging powers with alcohol, and suffers from increased blood pressure, is as much the victim of the conditions created by present-day methods of living as is the collier whose lungs are slowly being destroyed by the dust of the mines in which he works. The pampered woman, who, from sheer boredom, develops bad health, and the over-driven factory worker who lacks fresh air and leisure, are equally the victims of a wrong technique of living. Their recovery entails a complete alteration of their mode of life and a return to a more natural existence. More often than not this is as impossible for the rich as it is for the poor. Those who have grown up with the belief that a clever manipulation of money, or a prominent position in society, are the be-all and end-all of existence, have as many difficulties in finding a new orientation in life as the underpaid worker struggling to survive on inadequate earnings. Neither can follow the doctor's advice to 'change their mode of life', and both serve to illustrate the truth of the statement that the diagnosis of an illness is often easy, but the treatment of it exceedingly difficult.

The regulation of a patient's activities is usually an important part of medical treatment. Generally speaking, illness is an indication for a reduction of a patient's activity, either of his total activity or of that organ or structure which is principally affected. As a rule the need for rest is known to the sick organism instinctively; the ailing animal creeps into a quiet part of the wood to lie down, and the sick man naturally takes to his bed. Pain utters its sharp note of warning, the guardian muscles contract, and the inflamed joint is kept rigidly immobile. This cessation of all unnecessary activity is one of our most potent methods of treatment. Stephen Paget, a noted nineteenth-century surgeon, entered the lecture hall at St. Bartholomew's Hospital to lecture on the treatment of inflamed joints. He looked at his audience and addressed it as follows:

> Gentlemen, the first point of importance in the treatment of inflamed joints is rest, the second point is rest, the third is rest. Gentlemen, that concludes my lecture for to-day.

He then bowed and left the lecture hall. The splinting of broken limbs, the giving of pepsinized milk and of easily digestible fluids to patients suffering from gastric disorders, the use of dark and quiet rooms for cases of concussion, the ordering of plaster waistcoats and invalid carriages for tuberculosis of the spine, and of digitalis for failing hearts are all instances of the application of this general principle that a diseased structure must be kept at rest.

A mere cessation of activity would be of little value were it not for the fact that, given favourable conditions, diseased structures tend to recover. Doctors act only as the collaborators of that great physician, the body, and sometimes all we have to do is to keep our patient quiet and cheerful until it has completed its work. At other times we are able to aid our patient's efforts by administering some simple remedy.

The opposite form of treatment, namely, the increasing instead of the diminishing of activity, is sometimes called for. It is a physiological law that prolonged disuse leads to deterioration of structure; muscles that are never contracted grow flabby, lungs which are not fully expanded lose their elasticity, joints that are kept immobile stiffen, the circulation in a disused organ tends to become sluggish. Activity is essential to health, for as we have seen, nothing in the universe can remain stationary; it must increase or diminish, grow or die. It is on account of their stimulating action on sluggish organs that the various forms of physio-therapy, graduated exercises, electrical stimulation, medicinal baths and massage are of service to the sick. If men lived healthy natural lives, the use of these remedies would be very restricted and they would only be employed to counteract the effects of an enforced rest, to restore, for example, the atrophy of muscles following the breakage of a limb, or the loss of vascular tone, which is the result of a prolonged stay in bed. But because many of us live an entirely unnatural existence in towns and cities, these artificial methods of stimulating inert tissues are of great service to us. A lady of immense wealth and weight known to the writer found it pleasanter to keep a Swedish masseuse resident in her house than to dispense with her Rolls Royce. Massage saved the situation, but unfortunately the high standard of luxury in the house proved the undoing of the masseuse. She also became in need of similar aids to degenerating muscles and to a sluggish circulation.

The main benefit to be derived from a visit to a spa does not come from the salts dissolved in its medicinal springs. At Carlsbad or Matlock, a patient not only drinks water, but willingly submits to a discipline that could not be enforced in his own home. His diet, his daily exercise, his hour for retiring and rising, his alcoholic intake and his daily consumption of cigars, are all brought under review, and, tamed by the example of others, he agrees to their being regulated. Exercise, discipline, fresh air, dieting and a healthy action of the bowels soon begin to work wonders, and after a few weeks of healthy living, the patient is enabled to return home, and to carry on until the month for the annual spring cleaning of the body comes round again. The full effects of the waters of Carlsbad and Matlock can never be bottled; they must be drunk bubbling and gaseous at their source, for it is the regime of 'taking the waters' and not the actual waters that confers the greater benefit.

This method of treatment is as old as the civilization for which it is a remedy. Langdon-Browne, in describing medical treatment in ancient temples of Aesculapius, states that Greek doctors relied almost entirely on the use of hygienic and psycho-therapeutic measures. Built on the brow of some Grecian hill, the temples of Aesculapius were ideally placed to act as centres of healthy living.

> The ordinary hygienic measures ordained by Aesculapius were cold bathing, bleeding, anointing with mud or sand, walking with bare feet, exercise in the open air, and riding.

What could be better for the Greek patricians sated with the pleasures and refinements of Athens than the regime prescribed by the temple physicians? The same excellent methods, with certain minor adjustments, are now being used in the watering-places of Europe. The only changes which have been effected have been the replacement of bleeding by electrical treatment and massage, and, for the oracular pronouncements of priests, the substitution of positive suggestions of health from the lips of highly qualified physicians. As in the temples of the ancient world, so in our modern hydropathics, reliance is placed on hygiene tinctured with suggestion.

The patient who is under the necessity of making an annual visit to a spa in order to correct the results of wrong living is really a man who has violated his own bodily instincts. Deep within him he knows how he should live, for the body, as well as the mind, has its own criterion of sanity. Primitive man, like the animals, generally knows what is good for him, what food he requires, and how much rest is necessary for recuperation, and primitive man is generally guided by his instincts. Unfortunately civilized man has lost much of his natural wisdom, and even if it sometimes speaks to him he often turns to it a deaf ear. But as a rule the man with a low blood-sugar content instinctively craves for sweets, and Oliver Wendell Holmes tells us that the scurvy-stricken sailor of the past instinctively 'snuffed up the earthy fragrance of potatoes, the food which was to supply the elements wanting to their spongy tissues' This being so no doctor is ever wise to dismiss lightly the innate desires of his patients, even although these may seem to run counter to his own professional theories. When he does so he generally makes an error, as was the case when doctors treated high fever by depriving their patients of the fluids for which they clamoured. Fortunately medical men have now recognized that this was an error, and not only give their patients drink, but have substituted fresh air and sponging for overheated and airless rooms. Nor should the voice of the body be entirely ignored, even when it asks insistently for food which theoretically seems unsuitable. I can remember an ailing old lady who loudly demanded lobster for supper, and when at last she was allowed to have her way, consumed her meal with relish and impunity. In medicine as in other departments of knowledge an ounce of practice is worth a pound of theory.

It will have been noted that Greek practice made little use of medicines; they are nót even mentioned in Langdon-Browne's summary of the treatment employed in the temples of Aesculapius. Medicines were introduced by the Arabian doctors of Alexandria and, at a later date, were extensively employed in Rome. Dioscordes, a surgeon in Nero's army, is reputed to have compiled the first pharmacopoeia. Attached to one of the Roman legions, he made a practice of collecting particulars of the medicinal herbs which were used in the different countries through which the Roman army passed. It was from his pioneer work that the celebrated Galen afterwards derived his knowledge of drugs. Galen was a man of great eminence and a skilled physician, but with the decline of learning and the coming of the dark age to Európe, the giving of medicines no longer remained in the hands of men of this character. Drug pedlars attended fairs in the towns and sold to the crowds love-philtres and curative herbs, whilst witches and wise women in the rural districts brewed concoctions for their private clientele. But ignorant though these non-medical purveyors of medicine were, we owe to them many of the remedies which are employed at the present day. Digitalis is an example of a drug which was derived from the early herbalists, who used it in the form of a decoction of foxglove leaves. Naturally, a great deal of superstition was attached to the giving of drugs, and, speaking generally, the greater the rarity of the medicine prescribed, the more it was prized. H. W. Haggard quotes from a letter written in 1595, which gives details of the treatment prescribed to Queen Elizabeth's ambassador at the court of Henry IV. This letter states that

> the King's physicians gave him Confectio Alcarmas, compounded of musk, amber, gold, pearl and unicorn's horn, with a pigeon applied to his side, and all other means that art could devise.

In addition to these rare remedies, powdered mummy was much in favour, mainly because mummies were difficult to come by.

It was only in the nineteenth century that the various drugs used by physicians, apothecaries and herbalists were submitted to scientific scrutiny. This critical examination resulted in a complete revision of the pharmacopoeia and the elimination of many drugs that were believed to be either inert or harmful. The work of surveying all the ancient recipes proceeded slowly and, as was to be expected, many differences of opinion were expressed as to their value. What made agreement more difficult was the fact that the medical profession was uncertain what it was looking for, and what action was desirable in order that a drug should be deemed helpful in the curing of a disease. The majority of doctors were of the opinion that medicines must counteract the symptoms produced by the illness; if the heartbeats were quickened, digitalis should be given in order to diminish their frequency; if the temperature were raised, an antipyretic must be administered. But now arose a new and contradictory school of thought, the homoeopathic school headed by Hahnemann. These homoeopathic doctors pointed out that as symptoms were the result of the body's effort to overcome the disease, they should be reinforced rather than weakened. Physicians were there to assist, not to render more difficult the body's struggle to recover. The homoeopathic school of medicine laid down a new principle, namely that illness should be treated by giving drugs which produced similar effects, a principle which was crystallized in the dictum, similia similibus curantur' (like is cured by like). On a priori grounds there is much to be said in favour of this view. It must, however, be borne in mind that things which are similar are not necessarily identical, and that in prescribing a drug which seems to produce symptoms resembling those caused by a disease, the homoeopathic doctor may be acting like the Hindu who treats his jaundice by painting himself a brighter yellow with tumeric. Nevertheless, the basic principles of homoeopathy would seem to be sound, and allopaths, or those who treat like with unlike, actually subscribe to the homoeopathic doctrine in certain forms of treatment. Vaccine therapy is an excellent example of a remedy used by allopaths which acts by provoking symptoms which are similar to the disorder. As in so many other cases of a difference in opinion, it is probable that truth lies between the two rival schools of thought. If it be the object of a physician to exercise some sort of control over the body of his sick patient, he must be prepared to employ both methods of treatment, sometimes reinforcing its reactions and at other times diminishing their violence. We have seen that certain illnesses, such as asthma, are due to an exaggerated response to a comparatively mild stimulus. In such cases it would be illogical to increase by means of drugs what is already excessive, and during the attack of asthma some form of allopathy is clearly indicated. When the attack is over homoeopathy may prove more serviceable. This indeed is the modern method of treating asthma. An exact diagnosis is first made, and the nature of the stimulus to which the patient is hyper-sensitive determined. Then by the use of injections of increasing strength the patient is gradually desensitized to the irritant which happens to be the cause of his trouble.

A belief in the curative properties of certain potions is innate in humanity and a therapeutic action has at one time or another been attributed to almost every substance that is at all unusual. Haggard reports that when the potato was first introduced into Europe and was rare and expensive, it was used as a medicine and not as a food. When the novelty attached to this vegetable had worn off, it ceased to have medicinal value and was regarded only as a food. This idea that an illness can be cured by the drinking of a magic potion has persisted through the ages, and even at the present day the belief is widely held that the giving of some drug is a necessary part of all treatment. The bottle of medicine, or the box of pills, are the modern substitute for the healing amulet, and few hospital out-patients feel that they have received their due unless they have been provided with eight ounces of pharmaceutical magic. Nor is the belief in drugs confined to the uneducated classes. Haggard reminds us that when Carlyle heard that his friend Henry Taylor was ill, he immediately went off to visit him, carrying in his pocket the remains of some medicine which had helped Mrs. Carlyle on the occasion of a recent indisposition. Carlyle did not know what was in the bottle, or what was the matter with his friend, and had even forgotten the nature of the complaint from which his wife had previously suffered. But the medicine which had worked in one case would surely work in another, and comforted with the thought of the aid he was bringing him, Carlyle hastened to his friend's bedside. This belief in the magical properties of draughts and pills is so widespread that it is small wonder that the patent medicine business pays big dividends. The companies which supply these nostrums have taken the place of the travelling apothecaries, who were such serious rivals to the qualified physicians of the sixteenth and seventeenth centuries. These pedlars of medicines caused so much embarrassment to the physicians that legal actions were brought against them; in France the lawsuits were settled in favour of the physicians and in England in favour of the apothecaries.

The beginning of the twentieth century witnessed a new and revolutionary departure in the drug treatment of disease. Hitherto the various preparations in the pharmacopoeia had been used empirically, their value being judged by the results which were obtained. The year 1909 is an important one in the history of medicine, not so much because it was the year in which salvarsan was discovered but because it inaugurated a new method of discovering drugs. A few years previously Ehrlich, a German chemist, had expressed the opinion that there existed a specific for every disease, and that chemistry was the means by which it could be found. To prove his thesis he embarked on a search for a specific for syphilis. Starting with arsenic, which had for some time been used in the treatment of this disease, he made a large number of organic compounds, in the hope of finding one which would kill the spirochaetes of syphilis without injuring the patient's tissues. In 1909 he announced the discovery of a compound which seemed to answer his requirements. This he called salvarsan, or 606, this figure representing the number of experiments he had made in the course of his research. The year 1909 is therefore notable in medical history, because during it a chemist for the first time succeeded in synthesizing a drug expressly for the purpose of curing a definite disease. Stimulated by Ehrlich's success, many chemists have since worked along the same lines, with the result that we now possess a number of synthetic remedies (606, 914, M. & B. 693, 710, etc.) of the greatest value in the treatment of amoebic dysentery, sleeping sickness, puerperal fever, pneumonia and streptococcal infections. Each year adds to the list of valuable drugs so obtained, and although many diseases still remain unconquered, steady progress is being made.

But in the discovery of 'specifics' for various microbial infections there lies a certain danger, the danger of patients being treated by rule of thumb. As the old physicians used bleeding and purging as routine methods of treatment, so is there a risk of modern doctors employing the new specifics as a kind of panacea. Again the individual patient may be in danger of disappearing, and treatment be narrowed down to a conflict between the doctors and a certain variety of organism. It must be remembered that a medical man can never be a doctor to living things in general; he cannot even be a doctor to the human race. He can only attempt to help a single patient suffering from a disorder the exact nature of which is determined by his own innate and individual idiosyncracies.

In olden days, when medicine was in closer touch with philosophy and religion, it was said that where evil existed, nearby would be found the antidote to it; malarial fever existed in swamps, but in the same swamp God had conveniently planted the quinine bush, with its anti-malarial properties. On the basis of this idea, doctors sought for a remedy for rheumatism, an illness which was known to be prevalent in low-lying and damp districts. It was noted that the willow tree grew abundantly.in this type of country. Salicylic acid was eventually extracted from willow, and was found to be the best of all known remedies for rheumatism. Later ethyl-salicilate, or aspirin, was made out of salicylic acid by the chemist, and this drug to some extent sup-planted its predecessor. Applying the same principle, we can say that if organic life be the source of disease in human beings, there also in organic life may be found the antidote to it. From the very beginning of medicine man has instinctively taken this view, and has searched amongst plants for the remedies that would cure his illness. In taking this line doctors and herbalists have acted reasonably, for the basic chemistry of life is the same, whether it be the life of a plant, an animal, or of a man. Recent work on viruses shows that plants and animals may even be subject to the same diseases. For example, investigators in Japan have found that the virus of the 'rice stunt' disease, hitherto believed to multiply only in plants, can also live on insects. Researches in the United States have discovered that the same is true of 'Aster yellow' virus.

Although doctors have generally looked in the direction of the plants for their remedies for disease, they have sometimes searched amongst the animals and out of this has grown the science of organo-therapy. In all probability organo-therapy originated from the initial belief that by eating the organ of an animal the characteristics of that animal would be acquired. Courage would be obtained by consuming the heart of a lion, digestion aided by eating the stomach of an ostrich, and the poison of snake-bite cured by applying to the wound the body of the snake which had caused it. Crude as these old ideas may have ·been, they have in the end given results of immense service to mankind. The stomach of the ostrich contains a rich store of pepsin, which can now be extracted and given in the form of glycerine of pepsin, and although we make no use of the bodies of snakes in the treatment of snake-bite it is now known that the snake's immunity to its own poisons is due to the presence in its body of antibodies. The ancient saying that where evil is, there also will be found the antidote to it, has in many ways been justified; in organic life lies not only the cause, but often the best available remedy to disease.

The line of attack on disease adopted by preventive medicine is to carry warfare into organic life itself and assault those components of it which are hostile to man. The draining of swamps infested with malarial mosquitoes, the periodic stoppage of irrigation in Egypt in order that the snails which carry bilharzia may die of drought, the cutting down of reeds which harbour the fly of yellow fever, the slaughtering of rats responsible for the spread of bubonic plague, and the destruction of typhus-infested lice, are all instances of it. A striking example of man's warfare against a component of organic life which is hostile to him is provided by the fight which was waged against a new malaria-carrying mosquito introduced into Brazil from West Africa in 1930. That year a malignant form of malaria suddenly appeared in the neighbourhood of Natal (Brazil), which was recognized as being similar to that found on the west coast of Africa. Research by entomologists revealed the presence of a new mosquito, the *Gambiae*, well known in West Africa, but hitherto non-existent in Brazil. Since the maximum flight of this mosquito is three miles, it was concluded that the invader reached Brazil by means of the new air line recently established between that country and the west coast of Africa. The Public Health authorities of Brazil had been provided with an exceedingly difficult problem, for the *Gambiae* was a mosquito far more difficult to eradicate than the ordinary *Anopheles*, which had hitherto been responsible for malaria in Brazil, since it preferred to breed in tiny patches of water rather than in ditches and ponds. This prevented the use of a valuable method of combating mosquitoes, the introduction of a small minnow which feeds on its eggs and larvae. The danger of the new malaria carrier spreading over the whole of Brazil was great and an energetic campaign was organized against the marauders. Every possible breeding-place was treated with Paris Green, houses were visited by workers armed with spray guns, and all vehicles crossing from the infected to uninfected areas were stopped and fumigated. After immense labour and the expenditure of many millions of dollars, the danger to Brazil was finally averted, and the new mosquito was stamped out.

As more primitive men with their spears and their traps destroyed the carnivorae which preyed upon them, so does modern man, armed with scientific knowledge, reduce the number of his enemies amongst the simpler organisms of organic life. It would be possible to carry this analogy between the methods employed by barbaric and by scientific man still further. As primitive man enlisted the help of some of the more friendly animals, such as the horse and the dog, in his fight against his enemies, so does scientific man seek allies in organic life against disease. The use of minnows in the fight against the malarial mosquito is one instance of this. We also train other unicellular organisms to assist us in the destruction of pathogenic bacteria. Yeast preys upon the *staphylococcus aureus* (the organism responsible for boils and carbuncles), and yeast is now being used as a defence against these diseases. Moulds are the hereditary enemies of bacteria, and we are now beginning to use them as allies in our fight against different kinds of pathogenic organisms. The modern bacteriologist first selects the mould which he believes to be the most suitable for his purpose, and then trains it to attack the particular organism which is responsible for the patient's illness. He grows the most suitable mould lovingly in his culture tubes, pits it against the enemy, and when it has learnt to do what is expected of it, he utilizes it for treatment. It is probable that other friends in the great aggregate of life will later be recognized, and offensive and defensive alliances made with them. From organic life has come the illness, and from organic life likewise comes its cure. Where evil is, there nearby will be found its remedy.

CHAPTER II

SURGERY

SINCE the discovery of anaesthesia and of asepsis surgery has made such rapid progress that it has gained for itself an honoured place amongst methods of treatment. The art of the surgeon is almost as old as that of the physician, and in ancient Chinese manuscripts we read of famous craftsmen who undertook intra-cranial and intra-abdominal operations. It is, for example, recorded that Hua T'o, who was born in the first century after Christ, removed the spleen from patients rendered insensitive by means of a drug. But China was so remote that it exerted little influence on European thought. In the Greek school of medicine the surgeon was of no account, although Hippocrates wrote about wounds in the head and gave an excellent account of the treatment of fractures and dislocations. During the Roman Empire the surgeon became of greater importance since it was he that was called upon to cope with the ravages of the numerous wars in which Rome as a military power was engaged. Celsius, who lived in the reign of Tiberius Caesar, developed the new art and gained a great reputation by operating for stone, cataract and rupture, and by performing Caesarian section in cases of obstructed labour. After the fall of the Roman Empire the practice of surgery again declined, until it was eventually revived by Ambroise Paré. This great man learnt his craft on the battlefields of the sixteenth century, thereby supporting the view of Hippocrates that 'War is the only proper school for the surgeon'. Many years later another eminent army surgeon, Larry, Napoleon's own surgical adviser, studied in the same hard school of war, and during the bloody battle of Borodino, he performed as many as two hundred amputations a day. But these great army surgeons were not really representative of the men who were mainly responsible for the surgery of the sixteenth, seventeenth and eighteenth centuries Operating, like the dispensing of drugs, provided a living for a number of brutal and ignorant men, known professionally as cataract-couchers, lithotomists and booth-surgeons. Garrison quotes the complaint of William

Clowes, Queen Elizabeth's private physician, that surgeons were no better than runagades or vagabonds ... shameless in countenance, lewd in disposition, brutish in judgement and understanding'. These were the early members of the profession to which I have the honour to belong.

In former days the surgeon acted on the instructions of the physician who, being an educated man with a university degree, and the lineal descendant of the priest-physicians of Egypt, was the undisputed leader of the medical profession. The rapid advances that have been made by surgery since the discovery of asepsis and of anaesthetics have led to a change in the social status of the surgeon, and he is no longer the servant, but the colleague of the physician. It may be that the improvement of the surgeon's position has proceeded too far, and that his rewards are now out of proportion to those of the physician. If this be the case, it can easily be explained by the dramatic value attached to surgery, which makes such a strong appeal not only to laymen, but also to doctors. I can still recall my own feelings when as a student I watched the preparations for a night emergency operation at the hospital: the brightly lit theatre, the laying out of sterilized towels, the glistening instruments being lifted from the sterilizer and the patient wrapped in red blankets and lying on a stretcher in the dim anteroom, all made up a scene which was like the opening of some great theatrical drama. Then came an intensely exciting moment, the arrival of the great man from Harley Street. A short conference with the house surgeon, a few precise orders, the placing of the anaesthetist's mask over the white face, and a new act of the drama began. To me the man who now took the centre of the stage seemed a being from another world, a being with miraculous power, who could decide the issue of life or death. And he took it all so easily, his hands moving with the quickness and precision of a skilled cabinet-maker, his face expressing none of the emotions which I was feeling. I longed to become like the great dispassionate man working under the fierce light of the operating lamp.

Yet if the profession of physician and of surgeon be considered detachedly, there cannot be the slightest doubt that the work of the physician makes greater demands for skill and knowledge than does that of the surgeon. There are many great surgeons, but few really great physicians. Not only must the physician possess a wider range of knowledge, but he must also be endowed with that indefinable faculty usually called intuition, which gives him an almost clairvoyant understanding of his patient. A surgeon can be made because he is a craftsman rather than an artist, but a true physician must be born. This does not mean that a good surgeon can be entirely lacking in the special qualities which are essential to the making of a physician. If he is merely a craftsman who by patience and devotion to his work has acquired a good technique, he will never be a good surgeon. A dexterous handling of instruments is not enough. There are some brilliant technicians who, because they can look inside a patient's abdomen and leave only a neat scar as a souvenir, show no hesitation in advising an exploratory operation whenever a precise diagnosis is in doubt. Because they are essentially materialistic in their outlook they are totally unaware of the psychological trauma which an operation may inflict on the mind. Such surgeons think only in terms of mechanism, of removing, sewing up, making anastomoses between one organ and another or of freeing the passages from obstructions. Preoccupied with the machinery of the body they forget about the existence of the mind and spirit.

It is interesting to study the wide range of reactions shown by different patients to the idea of an operation. To some people the news that they must be operated upon comes as a severe shock. They are overwhelmed by morbid fears, sometimes connected with the operation, and sometimes with the anaesthetic, for it is not everyone who is willing to lose consciousness and leave his body in the hands of another to do that with it which may seem necessary. I can recall one patient who received the news that an operation was unavoidable with complete calm, but who when told that it must be done under an anaesthetic was thrown into a state of panic. He suddenly sat bolt upright in his chair and after a momentary hesitation, gave the explanation of his fear: 'I have had four anaesthetics in my life, three for teeth, and one for a small operation, and on every occasion I have met the Devil. I never want to meet him again.' Only after having been reassured that if suitable precautions were taken, and if avertin were given as a premedication, the intrusion of His Satanic Majesty would be prevented, did he consent to the operation.

In strong contrast to the panic-stricken type of patient are the patients who apparently derive some private satisfaction from the news that an operation is necessary. To such people the fact that they are to play the chief part in the drama of the operating theatre brings a feeling of enhanced self-importance, for the light thrown by a modern Zeiss theatre lamp upon the operating table is as dazzling as the fierce light which beats upon a throne. It is true that payment is exacted for being so powerfully illuminated, but this applies equally to kings; they also must make payment for the privilege of wearing crowns. But whatever be the precise nature of the satisfaction to be derived from having an operation, there are people who collect operation scars with the same enthusiasm as is displayed by a schoolboy collecting stamps. The scar experts have the special advantage of carrying their collections on their person, an advantage which enables them to exhibit prize specimens to all who have similar interests. This hobby is not necessarily, as might perhaps be thought, the prerogative of the idle rich. Abdomens are daily uncovered in the out-patient departments of our great hospitals which are stencilled with pale parallel lines, the handiwork of a number of different surgeons. The owners of these decorations are usually well-versed in medical jargon, and can narrate without faltering the symptoms appropriate to movable kidney, dilated stomach, dropped womb or distended gall-bladder. But there is a limit to all human endeavours, and Mr. X., Miss Y. and Mrs. Z. eventually become so well known in the local hospitals that they find it impossible to add new specimens to their collections.

The old suspicion that patients are enticed into hospitals in order that surgeons may experiment upon them is dying out, and I am deeply impressed by the quiet confidence with which the average hospital patient accepts the news that an operation is necessary. This confidence is all the more surprising when one realizes that the patient does not know, and but rarely asks to be told, the nature of the liberties which are to be taken with his body. There is something pathetic in this blind confidence of a grown person in the judgment of a man who is a complete stranger to him. But the trust shown by the hospital patient is not only a negative quality due to ignorance and inability to realize the situation, it also has positive ingredients, for the poor have often acquired a more realistic attitude to life than have the wealthier and more educated classes. They do not require a Carlyle to tell them that there is no such thing as security, and the labourer lying in the general ward of a hospital usually accepts the news that he has to have an operation in the same spirit in which he has accepted the innumerable difficulties he has already encountered, with a grumble, a jest or an inarticulate stoicism. After thirty years of hospital practice I have the greatest respect for the courage, the good humour and the patience of the men and women amongst whom I have worked.

Only exceptionally does a patient exact conditions before agreeing to an operation. The presence of the patient's family practitioner in the operating theatre during the operation cannot be regarded as a condition, for the family practitioner is a medical colleague who can often supply the surgeon with information of the utmost value in the taking of any decisions. But the presence of a relative, for example, of a parent in the case of an operation on a child, would rarely be tolerated. My old well-beloved chief, Sir Anthony Bowlby, told me that on one occasion he acceded to a father's request to be a spectator of an operation on his child for the removal of tonsils. The experience was not one that he wished to repeat. The father stood, robed in a sterilized gown, in a corner of the theatre, watching the final preparations for the operation. The induction of anaesthesia began whilst Bowlby was sterilizing his hands and putting on his gown. Suddenly the whole atmosphere of the theatre became tense, for the child had stopped breathing, and worse still, his face had become blanched. Without a moment's hesitation, Bowlby, who had seen the peril, quietly walked across to the operating table, took a firm grasp of both ankles with his left hand, held the child high in the air, and slapped its back vigorously There was a welcome gasp from the child and breathing was resumed. Quietly replacing the small patient on the table, Bowlby turned to the astonished father, saying: 'We always do that with children to encourage breathing whilst they are going under.' Little did the father know how nearly his child had died.

In the East strange conditions may be imposed upon the operating surgeon, sometimes without any previous warning having been given. A colleague tells me that when about to operate on an Oriental potentate, he heard strange music coming from a room adjoining that which had been prepared as an operating theatre. Unknown to him an orchestra had been installed there which supplied music during the whole of the operation. He never learnt why this was thought to be desirable. Another London surgeon narrates that on his arrival at a Maharajah's palace, having been summoned to operate, he was greeted by a venerable court official. This functionary inquired the date and precise hour of his birth. After this unexpected question had been answered, so far as it was in the surgeon's power to do so, the old man retired. Next day he returned and intimated that the preparations for the operation could proceed. He was the Court Astrologer.

It has been pointed out that the surgeon is a more romantic figure than the physician in the public mind. Novelists portray him as fearless and imperturbable, wielding his scalpel with consummate skill and absolute precision. 'One faulty movement, a moment's hesitation — and Death would seize his chance. . . .' The picture is a false one. Manual dexterity is not the most important quality required by the surgeon, even although it is an essential part of his equipment. The most vital requirement is good judgment and a capacity to make quick decisions. It is true that because the successes and failures of a surgeon are more apparent than are those of a physician, he is in need of greater confidence and boldness. But this does not mean that the surgeon can afford to be fearless. The ideal attitude has been summed up admirably by J. S. Mixter, himself a surgeon:

> A true surgeon is never fearless. He fears for his patients, he fears for his shortcomings, his own mistakes, but never fears for himself or his professional reputation.

It must be remembered that an operation is itself a confession of failure, a failure on the part of the body to regain its equilibrium, or of the physician to provide the help that it requires in order to do so. The ideal of modern medicine is to discover and treat diseases at an early stage, when pathological processes are still reversible, and the body can be completely restored to health. It is obvious that the later the stage at which the medical man intervenes in an illness, the less likely is he to succeed in achieving this ideal. Prolonged illness inevitably results in alterations in structure and to the development of conditions which are no longer reversible. Even if the pathological process be arrested, the body will have been irreparably damaged. Already better methods of diagnosis and more efficient treatment are leading to the avoidance of those conditions for which surgery is the only remedy. This can best be illustrated by reference to the modern treatment of digestive disturbances, and more particularly, of disturbances of duodenal digestion. It has now been shown that psychological factors have much to do with the development of duodenal irritation. The man who develops such digestive troubles is usually what is popularly known as a 'highly strung' individual, sensitive, anxious, and seldom relaxed either in mind or in body. If the emotional difficulties which predispose to a disturbed function of the duodenum are neglected, the illness proceeds to the development of an ulcer. The patient then passes under the care of the physician, who by rest, dieting and the use of alkalis, does his best to secure the healing of the ulcer. But by this time the pathological processes may have already progressed beyond the stage at which they were reversible, for even if the ulcer heals, it will leave a scar behind it. Should it fail to heal, or should it heal and the scar lead to gross structural changes in the duodenum or the stomach, the surgeon's help is required. A tangle which cannot be untied must be cut, and the surgeon is primarily a cutter of Gordian knots. The trouble which started as the result of an emotional conflict combined with wrong methods of feeding and of living thus ends with the performance of an operation on the body.

With the gradual improvement of medical methods of treatment, and the earlier intervention of the physician it is probable that there will be less need in the distant future for the skill of the surgeon; more and more knots will be untied and fewer and fewer will be cut. It is true that at the present day, more, rather than less, operations are being performed. The reason for this increase is that the art of surgery is still developing and continually finding new scope for intervention. But when the causes of disease are better understood and effective treatment is instituted at an earlier stage, recourse to surgery will become rarer. Already progress in the treatment of pyogenic (pus-forming) infections has cut short many inflammatory processes before they have progressed to the stage of forming abscesses. By the use of the new synthetic drugs the infective agents are killed and surgical intervention is no longer required. When that great day arrives, as almost certainly it will, when the cause of cancer is discovered, a still greater reduction will be made in the surgeon's work. Eventually he may become only the repairer of gross injuries caused by accidents, or the corrector of such congenital malformations as hare-lip and club-foot. The physician will then have regained the supremacy which he enjoyed during the Middle Ages, and will be recognized once more as the natural leader of the profession. Guirdham does not think that we shall survive even in a subsidiary capacity. 'Surgery,' he writes, 'is prone to piecemeal views and the fallacies of restricted vision. The surgeon of the future will in truth be a physician with manual gifts.'

The advantages which a surgeon enjoys are offset by a number of disadvantages. One is that his errors are more obvious and more severely punished than are those of his colleague the physician. All craftsmen are capable of doing bad work, but whereas the unsuccessful pictures of the artist are pushed into the back of the studio, the bad work of the surgeon is there to confront and disturb him. All his mistakes are not hidden underground. The twisted grimace resulting from the severed facial nerve, the halting gait of the badly set limb, the unsightly scar, the patient condemned to a life of semi-invalidism, all bear witness against him. Even when they have departed from hospital or nursing home his failures remain vivid in his memory, and from time to time walk like ghosts to disturb his peace of mind. If he be honest he is unable to lay them by disclaiming his responsibility. They are the result of his handiwork, and, if he has received credit for his success, he must shoulder also his failures. The surgeon plays for high stakes and must be prepared not always to win.

Occasionally, but surprisingly seldom, the surgeon is called upon to accept the unpleasing rôle of scapegoat. When relatives are facing the bitterness of beareavement they may be tempted to give vent to pent up emotions by finding that someone is to blame. If an operation has been performed, the surgeon is likely to be that person. He must be content to act in the capacity of scapegoat. He frequently accepts credit where but little credit is due; he must also accept blame where no blame is due. In doing so he performs a useful function.

CHAPTER III

PSYCHO-THERAPY

HEALTH depends on a state of inner balance and on a successful adaptation to environment, and since they are a unity the adaptation must be of the mind as well as of the body. The view that health is a question of balance is by no means modern. So long ago as 500 B.C. a Greek physician said: 'Health depends on harmony, and disease upon discord within the body.' Having considered the equilibrium of the body we can now turn our attention to that of the mind.

According to the catholic psychologist, Allers, man exists in four realms of being: as a physical being he forms part of organic life; as a human being he belongs to a community; as an intelligence he forms part of the realm of mind; as an immortal soul he belongs to the realm of the supernatural. Whether we accept Aller's schema or not, it is obvious that to be healthy a man must find adjustment in more spheres than one. This may be no easy matter. Unfortunately, man is not a unified and integrated being but a being in whom struggle for supremacy a great number of incompatible interests and conflicting emotions. He is 'a house divided against itself'. William James laid great emphasis on the incompatibility between the aims of man's various components. William James was no arm-chair speculator, but a practical psychologist who set out to find the 'self' by means of introspection, watching the stream of thoughts, emotions, sensations and memories which passed before him. Like the philosopher, Hume, he discovered that there was no true ego or 'self'. Instead he found a number of selves, a material self, many social selves, a spiritual self and something which he had great difficulty in defining, but which, from his description, would appear to have had many of the qualities of Bergson's 'memory' But it is of the conflict between a man's various social selves that he writes most vividly:

> Properly speaking a man has as many social selves as there are individuals who recognize him and carry an image of him in their minds . . . he has as many different social selves as there are distinct

groups of persons about whose opinion he cares. He generally shows a different side of himself to each of these different groups. Many a youth who is demure enough before his parents and teachers, swears and swaggers like a pirate among his 'tough' young friends. We do not show ourselves to our children as to our club companions, to our customers as to the labourers we employ, to our masters and employers as to our intimate friends. From this there results what practically is a division of a man into several selves; and this may be a discordant splitting, as where one is afraid to let one set of his acquaintances know him as he is elsewhere. . . .

And again:

I am often confronted by the necessity of standing by one of my empirical selves and relinquishing the rest. Not that I would not, if I could, be both handsome and fat and well-dressed, and a great athlete, and make a million a year, be a wit, a *bon vivant*, and a lady-killer, as well as a philosopher; a philanthropist, statesman, warrior and African explorer, as well as a 'tone-poet' and saint. But the thing is simply impossible. The millionaire's work would run counter to the saint's; the *bon vivant* and the philanthropist would trip each other up; the philosopher and the lady-killer could not well keep house in the same tenement of clay . . . So the seeker of his truest, strongest, deepest self must review the list carefully, and pick out the one on which to stake his salvation.

William James was impressed by the difficulty which a man made up of so many 'selfs' must encounter in reconciling the conflicting interests within him. Yet unless some adjustment be reached, no man can attain that harmony which we have seen to be essential to health. Physicians and surgeons are primarily concerned with the harmony of the body, but because man is not only a body, but also thought, emotion and consciousness, he cannot be treated merely as a biological unit — a plant. He is also a ghost. As has been previously said, it is impossible to sift out the factors in disease and state where the physical end and the psychic begin. The happy and the contented are more likely to remain healthy, and the depressed and the discontented to become diseased. No man ever caught a chill from wet clothes when enjoying a long exhilarating walk over the moors. Only when he is tired and dispirited does the cold and the damp begin to take effect. This is the earliest medical discovery I made. As a boy I resented my mother's insistence on the necessity for my changing my stockings when damp, and put my theory that this was all nonsense to a practical test. Running wild and by myself on the hills of Scotland I waded fully clothed in the burns, returning home in the evening after the wind and the sun had dried me, fortified and exhilarated by the secret knowledge that I had been right, and that no boy ever caught cold from wet shoes and stockings. Even that delicate and constantly ailing philosopher, Nietzsche, knew that contentment preserves one from catching cold. 'Has a woman who knew that she was well-dressed ever caught cold — No, even when she had scarcely a rag to her back.' (*Maxims and Missiles*.) Plato also was aware that the physical and the psychic in disease are so interwoven that it is impossible to separate them.

> This is the greatest error in the treatment of sickness that there are physicians for the body and physicians for the soul, and yet the two are one and indivisible.

Modern medicine has now arrived at the same conclusion, and psychotherapy has become an important part of all medical treatment. The unity of body and mind having been accepted, some of the classifications formerly used by doctors lose their meaning. The old divisions between functional and organic, psychic and somatic disease have ceased to have any meaning, for disturbances of function inevitably lead to changes in structure, and changes in structure to disturbances of function; prolonged emotional upheavals affect the body, and physical illness has its repercussions on the emotions. In future the terms functional and organic, psychic and somatic, will have to be regarded merely as convenient labels by which to indicate that in one case the functional disturbance is out of proportion to the structural lesion, and that in another psychic manifestations are more evident than organic changes; they will indicate the centre of gravity of the illness. And because there can be no organic disease which does not have some effect on the patient's 'psyche', all medical men will be compelled to study the main principles of psycho-pathology and psycho-therapy.

For the treatment of cases in which psychological symptoms are paramount special training and skill are necessary, and in order to deal with these adequately, a new type of physician, the psycho-therapist, has already come into existence. These specialists of the mind have done great service, but, as will be seen later, more must be asked of them.

When we look back into the past history of medicine how often do we find that later discoveries were long ago foreshadowed by some bold and original thinker who, because of his heterodoxy, was regarded by his contemporaries as a charlatan. Goethe once asked: 'Who can think of something stupid or something clever which has not been thought of by someone long ago?'—and Goethe as well as being a poet was a scientist. Towards the close of the eighteenth century Dr. Mesmer, an Austrian physician, wrote:

> to the physical causes of disease must be added moral causes: pride, ambition, all the vile passions of the human mind are as many causes of invisible maladies.

And then he asked:

> How can the effects of these continually reacting causes be cured?

At first Mesmer's metaphysical speculations merely amused his orthodox colleagues as is clearly shown in a letter written by one of them to a friend:

> At the moment Dr. Mesmer is creating a certain amount of sensation here, but actually he is only a little light, whom no one mentions except with contempt.

Later, when Mesmer attempted to find an answer to his question,

> How can the effects of these continually acting causes be radically cured?

his colleagues became very angry. Margaret Goldsmith describes in her life of Mesmer the reason for their anger:

> Rumours had reached the medical profession that, during some of Mesmer's cures, the patients were thrown into a very curious state of mind. They continued to carry out his instructions, they spoke and moved about, but they seemed, nevertheless, to be asleep, or at least unconscious of anything but Mesmer's person-

ality, his will. They were like sleep-walkers, so relatives of the patients reported . . . Mesmer's colleagues attributed it to witch-craft, or to activities of the devil.

Mesmer was evidently treating his .patients by the now well-known method of suggestion under light hypnosis, and what was more, was treating them with marked success. The sincerity of this early psycho-therapist, born a hundred years before the medical profession was able to receive his message, is reflected in his defence of his methods of treatment. In *A Letter to the Public* Mesmer wrote as follows:

> At present I have no intention of trying to convince anyone of my theories. I . . . shall not take up my time with controversy or pamphlets. Instead, I shall devote my time to my discoveries, from which the human race can expect to derive important and fundamental benefits.

Mesmer's expectations have now been realized.

Dr. E. B. Strauss says of psychology 'that it is the most abstracting (not abstract) of all sciences'. From the psycho-physical unit called man, a psychologist proceeds to make certain abstractions, which seem necessary to his requirements. One psychologist abstracts a number of psychisms which he calls instincts and which he does his best to define. Another selects other psychological phenomena which are termed variously temperament, personality, character and intelligence. So long as each psychologist uses his own abstractions empirically no difficulties are encountered. But when a number of psychologists meet together and attempt to synthesize their experiences into a single comprehensive system of knowledge, confusion inevitably results. This, to a great extent, explains the chaotic state of modern systems of medical psychology. As separate psychologies, and within their own framework, modern medico-psychological theories prove satisfactory, but they provide no firm basis for the creation of a general science of psychology. Freud's system of psycho-pathology is of value only in relation to the particular technique which he employed for the resolving of psychic conflicts. The terms 'the ego', the 'super-ego' and 'the id' are useful, but useful only in connection with the empirical method of psycho-analysis.

Briefly stated the aim of the analytical school of psycho-therapy is to extend the domination of reason and cognition into that region of the psyche which was previously controlled by unconscious motives. According to Freudian psychology a man is governed by his super-ego, a tyrannous form of 'conscience' existing in the submerged portion of his mind. This super-ego, however skilfully it may be disguised, is archaic, ruthless and superstitious, for it has been formed largely out of old impressions, old taboos and memories, and more particularly, out of the memories of important childhood figures, such as nurses and parents. It is a conscience which takes stock only of the lowest values, that is to say, of immediacy values. For example, a man ruled by his super-ego does not remain chaste because unchastity is incompatible with his religious aims. He does not make his choice deliberately, and with full knowledge of what it entails, but he is controlled by blind archaic forces, such as the muted voice which whispers in his subconscious mind: 'What would father and mother say if I were naughty?' He little knows that his actions are being determined by an out-of-date and tyrannous conscience expressing views which are perhaps at variance with his present mode of thinking. He does not live in a free and mutable present, but is chained to a fixed and immutable past.

Freud emphasized and, as most people now think, over-emphasized, the importance of the 'libido sexualis' in the genesis of psychic troubles. According to him, breakdowns in psychic adjustment generally arise from the fight between primitive sexual desires and the taboos imposed upon them by the primitive conscience. It was Freud's aim by means of analysis to effect a redistribution and a canalization of the affective charges derived from this sexual source. Adler, Freud's gifted pupil, came to the conclusion that his teacher was making too much of this conflict between sexual desires and the dictates of the 'super-ego', and substituted for it a conflict between man's natural instincts of self-assertion and the obligations which he feels towards the community in which he lives. Consequently in order to attain inner harmony it was necessary for a man to find his right relationship to society. Neuroses, according to Adler's view, were due to the individual's Will to Power failing to find social expression, and for this reason he called the new school which he founded 'The School of Individual Psychology'. Jung, a later and still more brilliant pupil of Freud, also broke away from Freudian orthodoxy, and taught that neuroses were the result of a breakdown in the mechanisms regulating a man's creative functions. In order to live harmoniously it was essential that an individual should find his own right mode of expressing himself.

Freud, Adler and Jung all made valuable contributions to medical psychology, contributions that were by no means incompatible or mutually exclusive. None of them evolved a method of treatment which is applicable to all forms of neurosis, but each made a valuable contribution to psycho-therapy. Medicine owes a great debt to all three of these great pioneers of treatment, and it is unfortunate that their disciples, and more especially the disciples of Freud, have shown more loyalty than judgment, and too often have bound themselves to a rigid and uncompromising orthodoxy. Fortunately a less fanatical school of analysts has now appeared which might be described as the eclectic and empirical school. The members of this empirical school make use of whatever method of treatment has been found to be of practical value, irrespective of its origin.

In order to be well adjusted in mind as well as in body a man's desires must not come into violent contradiction with each other, or run counter to public opinion, otherwise some of these desires are repressed into the more submerged part of the mind, there to produce a state of inner tension. The tension produced by this hidden conflict may lead to anxiety, obsessions and compulsion neuroses, or else manifest itself as disturbances in the working of the body, paralyses, tremors, pain or disorders of the various organs. Sometimes the manifestations of a psychogenic trouble change during the course of the illness, the patient who has hitherto displayed only psychic symptoms developing pain or disturbance of bodily functions. The shifting of the centre of gravity of the illness from the psyche to the body is generally associated with an improvement in mental balance and vice versa. For example, it has been found that if a neurotic patient becomes the victim of an accident, the symptoms produced by the broken limb may have a beneficial action on his mental condition. So frequently has this antagonism between mental and bodily troubles been observed that a new treatment of psychoses and neuroses has been instituted, namely convulsive therapy. By passing an alternating current through the frontal lobes of the brain convulsions can be induced in a patient suffering from mental symptoms. This often has a salutary effect upon the course of his illness. Why this should be so has not yet been satisfactorily explained, but it supplies yet another proof, if proof were wanted, of the closeness of the relationship between the mind and the body.

When the nature of the conflict is unknown to the patient, and is not revealed to the doctor by a superficial examination, a deeper analysis may be required. By getting the patient to pass into a state of reverie, thus permitting ideas to come up from the unconscious while the critical sense is in abeyance, the true nature of his anxiety may reveal itself. This in essence is the method of Freudian analysis, which is so largely employed at the present day.

However different it may appear to be, the rôle of the psycho-therapist in resolving psychic conflicts is the same as that of the physician in dealing with physical ailments. The aim of both psychologist and physician is to reinforce the natural tendency of the organism to regain its inner balance, and adjust itself to its environment. Whilst the physician is dependent for his success on the wisdom of the body, the psycho-therapist is equally dependent on the wisdom of the mind. At first sight it would appear that the body is more successful in correcting physical disturbances than is the mind in resolving psychic conflicts. Few patients fail to unite successfully a broken limb, but many do not succeed in healing the ills of the mind. But even the wisdom of the body has its limitations. When certain muscles are paralysed by an attack of infantile paralysis, unparalysed antagonistic muscles are liable to over-act, and to fix the limb in a position of permanent deformity. In order to guard against this physicians splint the paralysed limb, so that when it eventually recovers it may not be penalized by deformity. The mind may show a similar tendency to overact in psychological illness, and it is one of the psycho-therapist's functions to help the patient to avoid this exaggerated response to emotional trauma.

Psycho-analysis is undoubtedly a valuable method of treatment for cases of illness resulting from inner conflict. Whether the Freudian theory be correct or not, the treatment based on it provides the patient with the opportunity for giving vent to thoughts which hitherto he has been compelled to keep to himself. The mere fact that he has made certain confessions and that the analyst has accepted them as being not in the least unusual, or reprehensible, affords him considerable relief. Every patient is inclined to think that his own case is an exceptional one, and that nobody has ever been in precisely the same situation as himself. To know that this is not so, and that many people have overcome similar difficulties gives him encouragement. Analysis also helps a man to gain more self-knowledge, and this, we are told, is the beginning of wisdom. Not only does the patient become better acquainted with his own mechanism, but he learns to accept his peculiarities and to lose his feeling of guilt.

But although analysis may eliminate the conflict which has been responsible for a patient's illness, it has no power to help the patient to avoid difficulties in the future; it may restore him to health but does not teach him how to maintain his health. Having no orientation in life, no chart by means of which to steer his course, his condition remains precarious. Jung alone of the three great pioneers of the analytical school appreciated the importance of the possession of a positive philosophy of life if inner harmony is to be maintained.

> I should like to call attention to the following facts. During the past thirty years people from all the civilized countries of the earth have consulted me . . . Among all my patients in the second half of life — that is to say, over thirty-five — there has been not one whose problem in the last resort was not that of finding a religious outlook on life. It is safe to say that every one of them felt ill because he had lost that which the living religions of every age have given to their followers, and none of them has been really healed who did not regain his religious outlook. This, of course, has nothing whatever to do with a particular creed, or membership of a church. (C. JUNG: *Modern Man in Search of His Soul.*)

To reveal to a patient what was previously in the shadows, to show him more clearly the hidden workings of his mind, is, therefore, not enough. It may even lead to an increase of spiritual suffering unless a man be helped to find a philosophy of living. Who is to supply the patient with the 'religious outlook' which according to Jung he so sorely needs? Here is a difficult problem for which at the present moment there appears to be no solution. Freud was of the opinion that the finding of a way of life was the patient's own affair, and that for a psycho-therapist to foist on him his own beliefs was an unwarrantable intrusion. In any case, Freud was interested in neither philosophy nor religion, and regarded with considerable disfavour his disciple Jung's preoccupation with these subjects. He did not subscribe to the view that the possession of a philosophy or a religion was necessary to the maintenance of psychic health. He did not even realize that many of his own fanatical followers were converting his own teaching into a new religion, and him into a prophet, thereby showing that even after being analysed they had need of a religion and a 'father figure'. Nor did he recognize a parallelism in the bitter quarrels which broke out between his adherents and those of Adler and of Jung and the conflict which divides one section of the church from another. He was satisfied with his theories of the unconscious, and frankly admitted that he was not interested in religion.

Other psychologists, whilst less prejudiced against religion than was Freud, feel that it is not within their province to meddle with a patient's fundamental beliefs. Psychology concerns itself only with the temporal whereas religion and philosophy deal with the eternal, and many psychologists are of the opinion that by meddling with fundamental problems they may prejudice their search for truth within the boundaries of their own particular subject. In attempting more they may end by becoming not only indifferent philosophers but also bad psychologists. But the idea that a separation can be made between a man's method of dealing with emotional difficulties and his general philosophy of life is a vain one, and in practice it is found that the psycho-therapist who is attempting to help a patient finds that he is continually being drawn towards the threshold of philosophy and metaphysics. Sooner or later he is forced to cross it and to speak of ideas which are philosophical rather than psychological. And that it is his duty to do so is clearly the opinion of Professor William Brown.

> One cannot escape the philosophical aspect. One can help to disentangle things in a patient's mind — help him to see himself more clearly, and to realize how many of his motives are unworthy of him, and how unconscious mental processes are working in a repressed state of mind, and throwing up substitution forms in his conscious mind. One can show him the contrast between the conscious and the unconscious, and between the motives they reveal, and the more adequately that the psychologist

does this, the more successful he is, and then the more urgent it becomes to help the patient to a working hypothesis as to the meaning of existence and what he is in the world for.

The subject of the relationship between modern medical psychology and religion and philosophy is so important that it must be dealt with more fully, if for no other reason than that certain medical psychologists, as we have seen, have abandoned a neutral attitude to religion and look upon it as being synonymous with superstition. This is true of the great majority of Freud's followers, and in order to understand why this is the case it will be necessary to consider again their teacher's opinions.

Not content with having introduced a valuable method of treatment, Freud attempted to expand a working theory into a general system of psychology. In a book entitled *The Future of an Illusion* he seeks to prove that the Newtonian interpretation of the physical world around us is its final interpretation, and that human personality is merely a battleground on which blind desires wage war with the suppressive forces of self-interest, and with what he regards as being the illusions of religious belief. According to Freud a man's innate desire for something which is higher than himself, is nothing but the adult's substitute for the child's need for a 'father figure'; it is a redressing of infantile fantasies in theological apparel. He looked forward to the dawn of a civilization in which all religious superstitions will have disappeared, and in which science reigns supreme.

But Freud is thinking in terms of a science which has now disappeared, the materialistic science of the nineteenth century. His mind still lingers in an epoch when scientists believed that matter was something which was tangible and understandable, and that everything in the universe, from the falling of an apple to the writing of Shakespeare's Sonnets, could be accounted for by the working of mechanical laws. His physiology is of the same period, a physiology which attempted to explain life in terms of chemistry and physics. Since Freud studied these subjects as a student in Vienna, the whole trend of scientific thought has undergone a change. Scientists no longer look upon matter as being the one fundamental reality, or believe that the world described by the physical sciences is necessarily the only real world. And strange to say, it was the physicists who were responsible for the undermining of the elaborate structure of thought which nineteenth-century scientists erected on what they believed to be the secure foundations of matter. They did so when they declared that they had previously been mistaken about the nature of matter, and that instead of being solid and real, it turned out to be infinitely attenuated and elusive. They even began to use the language of the idealist philosophers, and to suggest that matter existed only in so far as the mind apprehended it, and that mind and spirit, and not matter, might turn out to be the ultimate realities. What words can be more redolent of Bishop Berkeley than those reported by the *Observer* to have been used by Max Planck when interviewed by J. W. N. Sullivan:

> I regard consciousness as fundamental. I regard matter as derivative from consciousness. We cannot get behind consciousness. Everything that we talk about, everything that we postulate as existing, requires consciousness.

What could be more idealistic in its outlook than the picture of the universe given by J. S. Haldane in the Gifford Lectures delivered by him in 1927 and 1928?

> The conclusion forced upon me in the course of a life devoted to natural science is that the universe as it is assumed to be in physical science is only an idealized world, while the real world is a spiritual universe in which spiritual values count for everything.' (J. S. HALDANE: *The Sciences and Philosophy*.)

The science. therefore, to which Freud looks forward as a means of freeing us from the superstition of religion, is a science which no longer exists except in the pages of obsolete books. And herein lies a strange paradox. Whilst physicists have been turning into Idealist philosophers, and physiologists have been developing a spiritual view of the universe, a large number of medical psychologists have been moving in the opposite direction. Physicists have found a place for spiritual values in the material universe and at the same time psychologists have asserted that they have no real existence in man; all else is spiritual and only man is material.

Because Freud made valuable contributions to medical practice and won a world-wide reputation as a psycho-therapist, his excursions into the realms of philosophy became invested with a spurious importance. He exercised a strong influence over the thought of the first thirty years of this century, and was acclaimed as a prophet by a generation which had been disillusioned of all orthodox religious teaching. Here at last was a gospel which it was possible for them to accept, a guide to living which they could follow. Repression came to be looked upon as a sin and the free expression of the unconscious as a rule of life. Many took Freud's message to mean that all moral standards were fictitious, and did their best to live in accordance with this interpretation Artists were encouraged to paint from the subconscious and produced subconscious works of art, of interest to students of psycho-pathology but having little bearing on art. Education, literature, painting, music and the drama were all in turn infected by Freudianism, and what had started as a working theory, applicable to a limited field of medicine, ended by becoming a pseudo-religion.

If it be true that the possession of a positive philosophy of life is necessary to the maintenance of inner harmony, a weighty responsibility rests on the doctor or psycho-therapist attempting to restore a patient's health. And it is a responsibility which few doctors will be willing to shoulder, for a doctor himself may not possess a philosophical outlook on life. Nor does his professional conscience trouble him if he has not been able to acquire one. At the same time he is usually unwilling to call in the help of the recognized professors of religion, the clergy. The medical suspicion of the purveyors of orthodox religion is not merely the result of professional prejudice, for a course of theology at an ecclesiastical college does not necessarily equip a man for the difficult work of helping a patient to find a new meaning in life. It may even prove a handicap to him, for more often than not, a clerical garb creates a barrier between a clergyman and a layman, a barrier which has to be broken down before they can talk freely. There are clergymen who are able to do this, and who quickly establish a sympathy between themselves and those with whom they come into contact, but there are others who remain only churchmen and the wearers of an unusual form of dress. So isolated do some of these clerical gentlemen appear to be from the rough and tumble of life that they create in those who talk to them the feeling that religion has no relationship to their private troubles.

Whilst a religious outlook is conducive to inner harmony it cannot be said that all who claim to be religious are necessarily blest with health. Guirdham reports that members of the more puritanical branches of Protestantism, such as the Plymouth Brethren, suffer much from melancholia and psycho-neuroses. 'Till I practised there (the West of England) I did not realize that people could die from that sense of guilt which inhibits the fulfilment of pleasure and destroys the psyche's rest.'

According to Prinzhorn, the ideal psycho-therapist would be a man compounded of

> one wise priest from each of the greatest religious communities, one lawyer, one teacher, one psychologist, one wise philosopher and three physicians possessing a very firm biological basis.

But where is this paragon amongst psycho-therapists to be found, this wise priest with a knowledge of science and possessed of a religion which transcends the narrow boundaries of church and creed? In the East the ideal blend of psycho-therapy postulated by Prinzhorn still probably survives, but in the West it is non-existent. From the beginning of its culture there has been found in India the cycle of sciences known as yoga, a system of knowledge which provides all that is necessary for the welfare of body and spirit. From Hatha yoga a man learns how to maintain and to increase his physical health, and by means of Rajah yoga, 'the kingly art', he is taught the control of the mind. Bhakti yoga is the yoga of religion, Gñani yoga is the yoga of knowledge, and Karma yoga the guide to right action. All that a man requires to know is to be found in this ancient system of knowledge, and if its help could be enlisted by Western medicine it would prove to be of incalculable value to it. But for several reasons this is impossible. In the first place, knowledge of yoga is unobtainable in Europe, for it is knowledge which can only be imparted by a teacher and can never be learnt from a book. In the second place, it is knowledge which, even if it were obtainable, is incompatible with Western ideals. To live according to the teaching of the yogis we should have to sacrifice all that we have learnt to prize most highly — material success, commercial prosperity and worldly power. No compromise is possible. A branch of knowledge cannot be isolated from Eastern thought and grafted on

142

to a culture which is entirely foreign to it. If this were attempted the result would be the making of a travesty of yoga in which there was nothing left which was capable of surviving. Finally, it has to be admitted that because of the backwardness of its medical sciences Western doctors would never think of looking in an easterly direction for knowledge. This indeed is true of others than doctors. All the efforts which have hitherto been made to draw together Eastern and Western cultures have failed mainly because they have always been undertaken in the interests of the Western outlook. Europeans tacitly assume that what the East possesses, the West also has in greater measure. The East is always adapted to the West, and never the West to the East. As a result nothing is ever gained. It is therefore impossible for Western doctors to avail themselves of the knowledge which exists in the ancient practice of yoga.

This does not mean that there exists a chasm between Eastern and Western thought which cannot be bridged. Even if it is difficult for a Westerner to become a yogi he can learn a great deal from the Oriental's attitude to life. Eastern and Western people barter the products of their industry in the market places of the world. Surely the time has come when with even more mutual profit they can exchange the products of the mind.

CHAPTER IV

THE TWO WORLDS

THIS book is the outcome of an effort to find an attitude to the problems of disease, pain, old age and death. It disclaims all pretensions of formulating a general philosophy of life. But it is obvious that the observations made in the consulting-room which are the subject-matter of this book cannot be treated as isolated phenomena, but must be related to some larger view. It is impossible to discuss the accidents of life without referring to the significance of life; it is impossible to describe pain and fear as instruments with which we have been provided in order that we may apprehend the dangers of our journey without at the same time considering the nature of that journey. However shadowy and incomplete the sketching-in may be, some indication must be given of the general background of this book. And of necessity it must be a philosophical background, because this alone will allow of the special knowledge which I happen to possess as a doctor being viewed in its proper perspective. Being a medical man and not a philosopher, my philosophy will be that of a practical man rather than that of a school dialectician, of a scientist rather than that of a metaphysician.

But I am of the opinion that in the end all philosophies are personal philosophies. They are the stories which individual men and women tell themselves in their attempts to explain the mystery of their existence. What form the story takes will, to some extent, be determined by the nature of the qualifications which the narrator possesses; the scientist explains his experiences by one kind of story, the artist by another, and the religious man by yet another, each contributing his quotum to the common pool of knowledge. Yet even those who tell the same kind of story differ in their manner of telling it, each adorning it with his own embellishments and giving to it an individual twist. As McNeile Dixon warns us:

> You can no more escape your philosophy than you can escape
> your shadow, for it also is a reflection of yourself . . . All reasoning

is in a manner biased, and the bias is due to the nature, surroundings and education of the thinker. (*The Human Situation.*)

Human beings are not built on the lines of calculating machines, which merely arrange and reassemble the material with which they are fed. Whatever we receive becomes our own, and on being returned is found to be stamped with the signature of our personality. This is true of all branches of knowledge, even of physics, the most developed of all the sciences. Sir Arthur Eddington has no illusions concerning the subjective nature of our knowledge of the physical world:

> We have found a strange footstep on the shores of the unknown. We have devised theories one after another to account for its origin. At last we have succeeded in reconstructing the creature which made the footprint. And lo! it is our own.

The mathematician who sets out to explore the universe finds that it can only be explained in terms of mathematics, the artist discovers that it was created by a great artist, the religious man, by a divine spirit.

Before sketching, in rough outline, the personal philosophy which forms the background to the ideas expressed in this book it will be helpful to discuss briefly the means by which all philosophies are reached. Man possesses two instruments of cognition; the intellect and the emotions. Through his sense organs he receives certain impressions, and by his intellect he interprets these and constructs from them various theories. His intellect is an instrument by means of which his experience can be formulated and given precision. It works in conformity with the laws of logic, and, as Bergson pointed out, is of great practical utility in the business of living. The emotions are equally an instrument of cognition, but an instrument which provides a different category of knowledge. Whilst the intellect deals with the material world of the senses, the emotions explore the unseen world of values. It makes no use of logic and is less concerned with the necessity of reconciling one view with another than with that of making a comprehensive sweep of the whole. Pascal gives an excellent description of the different approaches of the intellect and of the emotions to a problem.

> Those who are accustomed to judge by feeling cannot comprehend the arguments of logic, for they wish to pierce at a glance

the very core of truth; and are not accustomed to separate its initial elements, in order to reconstruct them. And those who by habit deduce principles cannot be convinced by the vision of pure feeling; they seek a rule, a law, and cannot be contented with a view.

In the emotions we have an instrument of great power and of immense subtlety, and, although its findings cannot always be clearly formulated, they carry with them great weight. So strongly indeed does a man feel the truth of his emotional discoveries in the world of values that they often appear to him to be of the nature of a revelation, of a message brought to him by some external agent. If, for example, he accepts St. Paul's words that 'the greatest of these is charity', and realizes the truth of the injunction: 'Therefore all things whatsoever ye would that men should do to you, do you even so to them', he does so with intense conviction, even although he may be unable to live up to the principles which they inculcate. Yet, when examined by the intellect, both these injunctions would appear to be not only impracticable but also unreasonable. Had it been the intellect which had formulated a workable code of conduct, it would probably have arrived at the conclusion that ill deeds must be followed by punishment, and that in order to survive a man must get the better of his neighbour. Instead of presenting his coat to another, a prudent man would be wise if possible to secure an additional garment. The intellect might admit that honesty is the best policy, but only as a means and not as an end. It would argue that a reputation for honesty always proves serviceable, but that excessive scrupulousness in business is often a handicap. The majority of the truths formulated in the New Testament are so different from those which the intellect would have arrived at, that they can only be understood, and then only partially, by some faculty which has the capacity to reach forward into the unknown, and intuitively grasp what lies outside the compass of argument. And because it is obvious that these truths could never have been discovered by the unaided intellect, the belief has arisen that they must have been revealed to a man from without. According to Christian doctrine, God had to take on flesh in order that the truths enunciated in the Gospels should be brought to earth. The conclusion that no ordinary man could have attained the knowledge which Christ imparted to His disciples is undoubtedly a true one, for the level of His wisdom was such that it could only have been reached by one in whom was developed, as in no ordinary man it has ever been developed, the germ of the divine within us. What is not usually realized is the fact that such a high level of wisdom demanded of those who heard it a higher level of understanding and a finer discrimination than the vast majority of Christ's hearers possessed. This is repeatedly affirmed in the Gospels, not only in the parable of the Sower, but also by the words which formed the prelude to so many of Christ's sermons. 'He that hath ears to hear, let him hear.' He spoke to the multitude only in parables, but to those who were being specially trained by Him, and who had left everything, homes, wives, children, occupation and possessions for the sake of their convictions, He expounded the real meaning of His teaching.

The statement that the emotions are an instrument of cognition requires amplification, for the term 'emotion' covers a great many different psychic experiences. From what is usually meant by the emotions, the petty cravings, jealousies, angers, and distresses which colour our thoughts and actions, can come no understanding. Instead of enlarging our field of vision, they narrow it until all that we can see is ourselves and our trivial grievances. It is only in those rarer moments when the spirit is unruffled by such unpleasant disturbances that it is able to reflect on its tranquil surface the image of truth. Then, for a brief while, we may be capable of feeling truths which previously were hidden from us. It is this faculty, akin to the creative vision of the artist, or the inspiration of the poet, called by Bergson intuition, which is capable of apprehending truth beyond the range of the intellect. But the contrast which has been made between the working of the intellect, and of the emotions, does not necessarily imply the existence of any contradiction in their discoveries. Emotional knowledge is not incompatible with the knowledge of the intellect. It is reasonable, but not ratiocinative.

Bergson has described the intellect as a faculty which presents us with an incomplete and fragmentary representation of the universe, and no better illustration of this could be given than that provided by the scientist's representation of the appearance of life on the earth. A scientist does not actually claim to account for this phenomenon, but he disguises his ignorance so skilfully that the unwary are led to believe that he has explained it. He states that the physical conditions on this planet became such that life was rendered possible. The environment being satisfactory certain complex molecules of matter organized themselves into those self-sustaining and self-reproducing energy-systems which we call life. By the interplay of blind forces the stage was set, and by the continued action of those forces, life came into being. Living matter, purposive, seeking its own ends, and accommodating itself to the forces around it, manifested out of the void. What a strange anomaly is this which the scientists would have us accept, this paradox that unintelligent forces should produce intelligence, that a purposeless universe should create a creature moved by purpose. And it is the purposiveness of life which is its distinguishing characteristic; life acts as though it desired to maintain itself, as though it were working to some plan. The purposiveness shown bv life, the ability of an organism to overcome difficulties, the capacity of the various parts to work for the good of the whole all make it impossible to explain life in terms of chemistry and physics. This the biologists now realize. To study the human body is to be filled with wonder. No machine, however artfully contrived, could repair its breakages with the skill with which the body makes good its injuries. Man's body can only be understood on the assumption that it is possessed of an intelligence which enables it to adopt those measures which are necessary for its survival. And what of man's mind? Has this also been born of the unintelligent universe? Bertrand Russell would have us believe so:

> Man is the product of causes which had no prevision of the end they were achieving; his origin, his growth, his hopes and fears, his loves and beliefs, are but the outcome of accidental collocations of atoms.[1]

Here is a typical product of the intellect, a cross-section of the universe which deprives it of all meaning. Russell himself appears to be struck by the anomaly which he has produced, for elsewhere he points out that 'it is a strange mystery that man can judge the work of his unthinking

[1] 'It is a strange mystery that nature, omnipotent but blind, in the revolutions of her secular hurryings through the abysses of space has brought forth at last a child, subject to her processes, but gifted with sight and knowledge of good and evil, with the capacity of judging all the works of his unthinking mother.' (*Mysticism and Logic*.)

mother Nature'. Strange indeed, but no stranger than many other incomplete or fragmentary views with which the intellect may present us. It is of course possible to maintain intellectually that the whole universe is meaningless and that intelligence is not in what is beheld, but only in the mind of the beholder,

> As a man thru' a window into a darken'd house
> peering vainly will see, always and easily,
> the glass surface and his own face mirrored therein.
> (ROBERT BRIDGES: *Testament of Beauty*.)

But this explanation only widens the gulf between intelligent man and the meaningless universe, and makes absurd demands upon our credulity. The difficulties which this particular method of thinking entails are as old as is the study of philosophy itself, and have been, in my opinion, answered best by Plotinus and by Zeno:

> The most irrational theory of all is that elements without intelligence should produce intelligence. (PLOTINUS.) Why not admit that the world is a living and rational being, since it produces animals and rational entities.' (ZENO.)

As human beings we can only interpret the universe in the terms with which we are the most familiar, the terms of intelligence, emotion, consciousness, will and purpose; we cannot see the world as a stone, or as a divinity sees it, but only as a man sees it. And we should be content to describe the universe as best befits us. But because during the last century physics was looked upon as being the basic science, and was held to make the closest contact with reality, scientists struggled hard to describe the universe in terms only of matter and force, on the assumption that this gave a more objective account of the outside world. This is an assumption which the majority of eminent twentieth-century scientists have now abandoned. Even the physicists, whose views provided the basis for the whole of nineteenth-century materialistic thought, have given up the idea that matter is the fundamental reality in the universe. The physicists have indeed so effectually destroyed the foundations of nineteenth-century thought that very little now remains of it. Professor Eddington goes so far as to state that the objects which physicists study are not constituents of the world in their own right, but symbols of real things, symbols which the physicists have constructed, and which reflect the interests and peculiarities of the minds of their makers. These symbols do not therefore bring us into touch with reality, and they only possess meaning in terms of each other.

The changes which have taken place in other branches of science, although less revolutionary than those which have been noted in physics, are very striking. How far biology has travelled since the days of Huxley will be obvious to anyone who reads the Gifford Lectures delivered by J. S. Haldane in 1929, from which the following quotation has been taken. Like Eddington, Haldane has discarded the language of matter, and chooses words which well might have fallen from the lips of Bishop Berkeley:

> It is thus only an imperfectly revealed spiritual world that we have taken for a material world; and so the world of our experience is a progressive realization of the spiritual world. This gives us a new conception of time, not as a mathematical entity, but as the progressive realization of one spiritual reality, involving space-relations as well as all other relations which make up an ordered world of values. (J. S. HALDANE: *The Sciences and Philosophy*.)

Professor Haldane may be right in postulating spirit, or consciousness, as the fundamental entity of the universe. Monism is the ideal towards which philosophers instinctively strive, but at the level of consciousness on which we move, such an ideal is unattainable. In whatever form the universe may reveal itself to the seer, the saint and the mystic, to ordinary mankind it appears in the form of a dualism. Since man first realized that neither he himself nor his world possessed unity, he has pictured his life as being a struggle between two opposing forces.

Man therefore appears to be living in two opposing worlds, the physical world of organic life and the unseen world of the spirit, each subject to its own laws, and each apprehended by a different faculty. Beneath the dualism lies some unifying principle, but to us who see only the surface of things, and that but darkly, the worlds of the flesh and of the spirit often appear to be opposed and contradictory. Inasmuch as we form a part of organic life we are committed to a ceaseless struggle, for organic life shows no mercy to the weak. To live is to struggle. The striving of marine organisms in a rocky pool, the surge of life in the soil and the clash of nations on the battlefield, all bear testimony to the bitterness of the fight in which all are engaged. When Christ said to his disciples, 'Ye have heard that it hath been said, An eye for an eye, and a tooth for a tooth: but I say unto you, That ye resist not evil; but whosoever shall smite thee on thy right cheek, turn to him the other also', he was pointing out to them an opposition between the two worlds. By no compromise could the few who had embarked on a new way of living expect to find peace; either they must continue blindly reacting in the physical world, or else put themselves under a different category of laws. No one could serve two masters.

In the foregoing chapters reference is repeatedly made to the conflicts in which man is engaged, the fight for physical survival and the struggle for spiritual development. Sometimes, as when dealing with illness, the emphasis has been placed on the fight for physical survival, and sometimes, as in the chapter on psycho-therapy, it is the spiritual conflict which is stressed. Occasionally both aspects of the subject have been discussed, for it is only by considering man's dual nature that he can be understood. If this be true of a man who is healthy, it is equally true of one who is sick. Medicine is slow in freeing itself from ideas which have now been discarded by science, but there are signs that doctors are realizing more and more fully that a sick man can no longer be treated only as a physical being. This limited conception of man was at one time necessary, and it has provided medical men with a good working hypothesis from which many useful and practical results have been obtained. It must now be abandoned, for neither the universe nor man can be explained in terms of matter, and a broadening of our view has become necessary. Our patients' minds have now thrust themselves upon our attention, and we can no longer leave them out of account even in the treatment of what appear to be purely bodily ailments.

Whilst psycho-therapy has already proved of immense service in the treatment of those illnesses in which psychic factors play the more important part, this new department of medicine has not yet had time to set its house in order. In spite of its enormous output of literature medical psychology lacks any generally accepted guiding principles, and because of this is split up into a number of different schools, which are not only in conflict with each other, but also with philosophy and religion.

There is also a certain danger in making psychiatry a separate branch of medicine even although this may be necessary for its progress. The patient's body and mind form a whole and it is impossible for the surgeon or the physician to hand over the mental symptoms in his patient's illness to a colleague as though they were subsidiary phenomena. The physical and the psychic factors in disease are inseparable and must be treated as one whole.

If we are right in believing that the universe has meaning and intelligence, and if Haldane's assertion that the reality behind the diverse manifestations of matter is a spiritual reality is correct, what then is the meaning and purpose of man? Because it is utterly beyond our powers to grasp the great plan in which the existence of spiritual beings finds some place, this question can never be fully answered. Herein lies a mystery beyond our powers of comprehension. Yet man seeks to know the unknowable, and in this very groping after truths beyond his ken, seems to reveal some purpose. Man with his limited mind seeks for the greater mind, man with his subjective vision seeks for the objective vision, man with his limited knowledge of good seeks for the source of all goodness. Man seeks for that which is higher than himself. What does it matter if his search be named differently by different people at different times; the search for the good, the true and the beautiful, or communion with God, Allah or Brahman?

The view which has been put forward that all the warring forms of life on the earth are but manifestations of a greater life, is not generally accepted by science, but has long existed in certain Eastern religions. To my way of thinking such a view would seem to be a necessary inference from any large-scale survey of illness.[1] It also falls into line with the trend of modern physics. The particle picture which depicts matter as consisting of separate electrons and protons fails to represent many aspects of the physical world around us, and recently there has been a disposition on the part of physicists to replace it by a wave-

[1] 'Just as the personality of a molecule is abolished in a crystal, so does the individual disappear in the evolution of organized beings, drowned in the mysterious stream which he contributes to form.' Lecompte de Noüy.

picture of matter. Commenting on this, Jeans states that although 'the waves of the picture are unobservable' it may be that a further study of them, rather than of electrons and protons, will lead us to the true objective reality behind appearance. (Sir James Jeans: *The New Background of Science*.) If therefore the physical world cannot be pictured in terms of separate and isolated particles of matter, if animal life can only be studied by relating it to all life, may it not also prove equally impossible to explain man's spirit apart from the existence of some greater spirit? In Drummond's *The Natural Law in the Spiritual World* a parallel is traced between the laws which control the phenomena in the two interpenetrating worlds in which man lives. I believe that the thesis which he expounded was right and that the fundamental principles underlying our existence in one sphere underlie also our existence in the other. If we knew more about the laws of the physical world we would also know more about the laws of the spiritual world, and vice versa. For the duality which exists between these two worlds is not an essential duality, but one which has been created by the limitations of our perceptions and understanding.

However different at first sight may appear to be the stories which scientists and religious men tell themselves, the theme which underlies them is the same. Looking at the vast surrounding universe, they see that it is in constant travail, for ever changing, for ever bringing forth new forms, and working towards the culmination of a plan so immense that it is beyond the power of man to comprehend it. From nebulae are evolved suns, from suns are formed planets, from planets satellites; all is a vast becoming. But the cosmos in which we live is not a completed cosmos, the dying universe of the Victorian scientist, but a universe which is in process of making. New forms are being evolved, old forms undergoing change and the whole of the mighty workshop throbs with the pulse of forces at work. All is a vast becoming. But as men, it is with the becoming of man that we are chiefly concerned. Whither is man travelling, and what is the fate which finally awaits him? In answering this question it is the religious man who speaks the more clearly and with the greater conviction. Man, he says, is engaged in a spiritual struggle for survival; either he will reach some higher plane of existence or else he will perish. The scientist speaks with less assurance, but having accepted Darwin's comforting thesis that an automatic evolution of man is already in progress, he generally assumes that man will develop to the fullest the intellect which is his pride and his distinguishing feature. The superman of the future will be a being of enormous brain capacity resembling the creatures which Wells's travellers found on the moon. But such a lop-sided evolution is more likely to lead to man's extinction than to his survival. Reason has not saved him from the disaster which threatens the civilized world, but has provided him with the means of destruction which he now finds himself to be entirely incapable of controlling. And it is these features which distinguish him from the animals and not his capacity for making tools and for manipulating for his profit the forces of nature that he must foster if he is to progress or even to survive. Bergson, to whose philosophy the views in this chapter are perhaps of all philosophies most closely allied, looked upon life not as a name which is given to a certain form of matter but as the name of a certain form of impetus. To him it is a visible current which passes from generation to generation, dividing and diverging and pushing against the inertia of matter until it reaches its most developed form. On many lines of its divergence the progress of the life-creating force has been arrested, or has even turned back on itself, but along the line of the arthropods and of the vertebrates it has found its highest expression. In the ants and in mankind are developed to the fullest degree two different forms of psychic activity, the instincts and what Bergson terms the mind. Wonderful though the functioning of the ants' instincts may be, these creatures are incapable of going further; they must remain for ever imprisoned in a mechanical perfection. But consciousness implies a limited degree of choice and to man alone, in so far as he is conscious, is given the capacity to create himself, not through the action of blind automatic forces but by never ceasing effort. With these views of the great biologist-philosopher I am in full agreement. Man is creation's furthest effort on this planet, man, the dimly conscious, man with his potentialities for spiritual development.

When man looks within himself he discovers there a conflict of interests, an incessant turmoil of forces, the antimony of good and evil.

Do you not see how necessary a World of Pain and trouble is to school an Intelligence and make it a Soul?

wrote Keats, and he was thinking not of the struggle for survival, but of the inner travail of the spirit.

I will call the world a School instituted for teaching little children to read — I will call the human heart the horn Book in the School.

The parable is a good one and as Keats says,

it does not offend our reason and humanity.

This is the oldest of all the stories which man tells himself in his attempts to explain the mystery of his existence, the story that the world is a school in which he finds himself working as a scholar, the story that it is a training-ground to which he returns again and again. And his scholarship and his training are not tasks which have been arbitrarily set him in a universe without meaning and without purpose. Intelligence and consciousness are not his alone, but are inherent in the very structure of the universe, his intelligence partaking of the nature of a greater intelligence, his consciousness of a greater consciousness. This is the story which I individually find to be the most realistic and the most satisfying. He is a microcosm of all that surrounds him, a universe in miniature.

In him proceed continual death and continual birth, the incessant swallowing of one being by another, the devouring of the weaker by the stronger, evolution and degeneration, growing and dying out. Man has within him everything from a mineral to God. And the desire of God in man, that is, the directing forces of his spirit, conscious of its unity with the infinite consciousness of the universe, cannot be in harmony with the inertia of a stone, with the inclination of particles for crystallization, with the sleepy flow of the sap in the plant, with the plant's slow turning towards the sun, with the call of the blood in an animal, with the 'three dimensional' consciousness of man, which is based on his separating himself from the world, on his opposing to the world his own 'I', and on his recognizing as reality all apparent forms and divisions. (P. D. OUSPENSKY: *A New Model of the Universe.*)

Surely this conception of man is more scientific, in the true sense of the word, than is Bertrand Russell's view of him that he is 'the product of causes which had no prevision of the end they were achieving'. Man has been fashioned out of the materials of the universe and there is everything in him 'from a mineral to God'. His fate is in his own hands. Either he partakes in ever-increasing degree of his spiritual inheritance, or he identifies himself more and more with the world of organic life, the world of fear, pain, disease, of suffering, confusion and death.

INDEX